EVERYDAY HOMOEOPATHY
A Safe Guide For Self-Treatment

Dr David M. Gemmell
MB, BS, BSc, MFHom

BEACONSFIELD PUBLISHERS LTD
Beaconsfield, Bucks, England

Supplied by
Ainsworth's Homoeopathic Pharmacy
38 New Cavendish Street
London W.1. (Tel. 01 935 5330)

First published in 1987

This book is copyright under the Berne Convention. All rights are reserved. Apart from any fair dealing for the purpose of private study, research, criticism or review, as permitted under the Copyright Act 1956, no part of this publication may be reproduced, stored in a retrieval system, or transmitted, in any form or by any means, electronic, electrical, chemical, mechanical, optical, photocopying, recording or otherwise, without the prior permission of the copyright owner. Enquiries should be addressed to the Publishers at 20 Chiltern Hills Road, Beaconsfield, Bucks. HP9 1PL, England.

© David M. Gemmell, 1987

British Library Cataloguing in Publication Data
Gemmell, David M.
  Everyday homoeopathy: a safe guide for self-treatment –
  (The Beaconsfield Homoeopathic Library; no. 8)
  1. Homoeopathy
  I. Title
  615.5'32   RX71

ISBN 0–906584–18–3

Phototypeset by Gem Graphics, Trenance, Mawgan Porth, Cornwall, in 10 on 12 point Times

Printed in Great Britain at the University Printing House, Oxford

Acknowledgements

I am happy to acknowledge my indebtedness to the following people for their valuable comments on the various drafts of the manuscript: Sue Allan, Michael and Lexi Barbakoff, Cornelia Navari, Dr Noel Pratt, Dr David Spence and Dr Jeremy Swayne.

Cathy Bolton typed the various drafts and I am grateful for her help and expertise.

I owe a great deal to my wife, Irma, for her encouragement. Our discussions about the design of the book and her editing of the various sections contributed much to its final form.

Finally, my thanks are due to John Churchill for his continuous support, encouragement and ever-elastic deadlines.

D.M.G.

Other Books Available From Beaconsfield Publishers

Classical Homoeopathy, Dr Margery Blackie. The complete teaching legacy of one of the most important homoeopaths of our time.

0906584140

Handbook For Care, Muriel Flack RGN & Margaret Johnston SRN. Practical guidelines for non-qualified people assisting qualified nursing staff.   0906584132

Herbal Medicine, Dr R. F. Weiss. Textbook of medical herbalism, with copious information on the clinical use of herbs.   0906584191

Homoeopathic Prescribing, Dr Noel Pratt. Compact home prescriber, with guidance on remedy selection for 161 common complaints and disorders.

0906584035

Homoeopathy In Practice, Dr Douglas Borland. Detailed guidance on the observation of symptoms and the choice of remedies.   090658406X

Introduction to Homoeopathic Medicine, Dr Hamish Boyd. A widely-used systematic modern textbook of homoeopathy.   0906584051

Materia Medica of New Homoeopathic Remedies, Dr O. A. Julian. Full clinical coverage of 106 new homoeopathic remedies.   0906584027

Nursing For Continence, Christine Norton SRN. Comprehensive text on the nursing care of the incontinent patient.   ·   0906584159

Studies of Homoeopathic Remedies, Dr Douglas Gibson. Major clinical studies of 100 of the most-used homoeopathic remedies.   0906584175

Contents

Contents

Contents

Contents

Introduction

Why this book has been written

Increasing numbers of people are becoming anxious about the severe toxic effects of many modern drugs. There is also great concern about the problem of addiction to prescribed tranquillisers, sedatives and pain-killers. Examples of such problems are almost certainly familiar to each of us.

Parents have become alarmed at the way that small children with recurring ear, nose and throat infections, and chest infections, are prescribed course after course of potent antibiotics. Catarrh is 'dried up' with drugs which at the same time not infrequently cause some degree of hyperactivity and sleeplessness. Older men may find that they have exchanged symptomless high blood pressure for a life of malaise, cold hands and feet, and impotence. Others will discover that the price of fast relief from the pain of rheumatism is severe indigestion, and occasionally ulceration and bleeding.

With all these problems there is a widespread feeling that we have handed ourselves over to 'the experts' – that we have lost the ability to participate in healing ourselves.

The development of modern scientific medicine has unquestionably brought enormous benefits to millions of people. But the price of overuse has often been the alienation of the individual patient from the medical profession, which, for its part, has been overwhelmed by the endless demands made upon it. People are also rediscovering that to acquire good health, and maintain it, they must begin to take responsibility for themselves and their families: 'You are part of the healing team – not a puppet or inert object of medical or surgical techniques. It is essential that you participate in your own recovery.' (Quoted from *Healing for Everyone – Medicine of the Whole Person*, by E. G. Loomis and J. S. Paulson, De Vorss Publishing Co., Marina del Rey, California, U.S.A.)

The first step towards acquiring and maintaining good health can only be taken by positive attention to diet, appropriate exercise, rest and relaxation, and the development of emotional and spiritual maturity.

The second step is to avoid the overuse of alcohol, as well as any use of tobacco and other drugs of addiction.

1

The third step is to appreciate that some illness is an inevitable part of life itself. Illness often indicates a lack of harmony in life as a whole.

The re-establishing of harmony may be achieved by attention to lifestyle, both short and long term, and by the use of various gentle and non-invasive therapies.

This is where homoeopathic medicine comes in.

Homoeopathic medicine works at different levels. It can be used by anyone for minor or short-lived health problems, even with limited knowledge or advice. At its most sophisticated, homoeopathy acts on the whole person and requires deep knowledge and much experience.

Homoeopathy provides a safe, inexpensive and frequently speedy method of treatment which can be used either in its own right or before turning to the more conventional treatments. It can be used on its own, or *in conjunction with* orthodox treatments. Homoeopathic medicine is complementary to all other forms of treatment.

This book is intended to help you and your family to use homoeopathy, at home and in safety. The problems I discuss are suitable for treatment by the reader. Wherever I feel it is essential to obtain professional advice, either initially or later on, this has been indicated.

If it is used as intended for minor health problems, you will almost certainly find that you need to call upon your own doctor's services less frequently. The fact that you have used homoeopathic remedies need concern him or her no more than if you had used any other self-help method.

It is important that you should have a National Health Service general practitioner, because sooner or later there will be a situation which will need orthodox treatment – such as surgery, accident care, expensive investigations or long-term support.

Take care to maintain the sympathy and concern of your NHS doctor by not demanding too aggressively that he becomes convinced of the effectiveness of homoeopathic medicine. It is a free country and doctors are as entitled to their own opinions as you are to yours.

Difficulties may arise when you ask to be referred to a homoeopathic doctor, or else to a homoeopathic consultant physician at one of the NHS homoeopathic hospitals (see pages 178–9). This usually arises when all orthodox approaches to a problem have failed. You have a natural and a legal right to have a second opinion, and if you wish that it should be from a homoeopathic physician, then that is your right too. But please be diplomatic in making your request.

Homoeopathic doctors have always worked within the traditional ethical framework of the medical profession, but have sometimes been frustrated by the reactions engendered in their orthodox colleagues by undiplomatic patients. Many general practitioners have recently become much more accepting of homoeopathic medicine, and it would be a pity to antagonise them with overenthusiastic or unrealistic expectations.

Lastly, I refer throughout the book to the 'doctor' or 'homoeopath' as being masculine. This is purely for simplicity and has no other implications.

What is Homoeopathy?

Homoeopathy is a system of medical treatment using medicine according to the principle of 'like cures like'.

As a theory and a means of treatment it was taught in Hindu writings over three thousand years ago. It was mentioned in the writings of Hippocrates in Ancient Greece. Galen described it in the second century in Rome. Paracelsus, the famous alchemist-physician, practised it in sixteenth century Europe. Throughout this long history the emphasis and sophistication have changed, but the principle has remained the same.

The principle is based on the observation that substances which cause symptoms can also be used to cure them. The homoeopathic method attempts to match the symptoms of a sick person with the description of the toxic effects of a particular substance. The same substance, in a much diluted form, can then be safely used as a medicine for the sick person.

It was a German physician, Samuel Hahnemann, who rediscovered the principle of homoeopathy around the year 1800. Hahnemann was one of the first doctors to research into the medicine of his day, using himself, his family and his students as guinea-pigs. The following facts emerged from his work:

- Overdoses of the common medicines then in use caused side-effects which could be recognised as distinct patterns of poisoning.
- Patients reacting individually to disease developed particular patterns of illness.
- It was often possible to match the pattern of the patient's illness with the pattern of the drug overdose observed in his experiments.

The next step was to treat the patient with the correctly matched drug, and note the frequency of successful treatment. Because of the strength of the doses that were then considered necessary, patients very often became worse before getting better. So Hahnemann diluted his medicines by stages in an alcohol and water solution giving them a vigorous mechanical shaking (termed 'succussion') between each stage of dilution. He discovered that these medicines were as effective as the concentrated ones but did not give rise to toxic effects. He also found that medicines prepared in this way remained medically active for several years.

Hahnemann experimented with the effects of many of the medicines of the time, such as quinine, and he also discovered the medicinal qualities of many new substances such as gold and silver. His successors in homoeopathy have continued to explore the use of many more substances, so that by now there are nearly three thousand of them. However, this little book is only concerned with about thirty remedies, because experience has shown that most common family illnesses can be helped by them.

Many examples of the homoeopathic principle in treatment are found in modern 'scientific medicine'. Generally they are unrecognised by patients as well as by the orthodox doctors who use them. For instance, X-ray overdosage can cause some types of cancer, whereas carefully controlled doses of X-rays can also cure some types of cancer. Amphetamines normally cause nervous excitability and physical overactivity, but a dramatic effect can be seen in the use of amphetamines for calming some hyperactive children. Another example is the use of vaccines in immunising against infectious fevers.

How to use this book
1) Look up the section you need (e.g. 'The Baby' – page 70). Alternatively, check the alphabetical Problem Index for the page number of your problem.
2) Turn to the appropriate page and read the left-hand page for the background information.
3) Read the right-hand page for the short description of the symptoms.
4) Compare these descriptions with the symptoms of the patient, and select the one which is the most similar.
5) Read off the name of the remedy suggested at the right of the chosen symptom description, together with the potency and the dosage scheme.

How to Select the Symptoms
As you use this book you will become aware that homoeopathic medicine aims to treat the patient as an individual and as a whole. What marks him as an individual is his own 'symptom picture'. The things which make his

symptom picture unique are his personal reactions to conditions like the weather, the seasons, the time of day or the way he is affected by movement or rest. His emotional make-up is most important too.

The Remedy

You will notice that some remedies will be suggested for several different and apparently unrelated conditions. This is because these homoeopathic remedies do affect the living processes in every part of the body and so are found to be medically active in many conditions. In other words, these major remedies are medicines for the whole person.

While it is important to take all the symptoms of a patient into account, this may in practice not always be possible: the purpose of this book is to show how even a limited view of the patient can help you to choose an effective remedy.

The remedies may be bought as pills, tablets, powders or granules. They are all made of lactose (milk sugar) and they have all been medicated in the same way with the liquid form of the remedy. The actual form makes no difference. Tablets are most commonly available: some may be harder than others and take longer to dissolve.

While pills and tablets are convenient for children and adults, powders are more suitable for babies. If powders of a remedy are not available, a tablet or a pill can be crushed between two clean, dry teaspoons.

Certain remedies are used in ointments or creams, and can be bought directly from chemists and health food shops. These remedies can also be used in solutions, and in this case are sold as alcoholic tinctures to be diluted with water.

Do not treat yourself with homoeopathic remedies if you are already being treated by a homoeopath. Check with him or her first unless the new condition is a simple one, such as using Arnica for bruising in a minor injury.

The Dose

In homoeopathic medicine it is not possible to be dogmatic about dosage and prescribing methods, because they are adjusted to each individual patient and his changing symptoms. Adjustments may have to be made following each change of symptoms.

One dose of a remedy consists of one pill, or one tablet, or one powder, or ten to fifteen granules.

Some manufacturers suggest giving one tablet for a child and two for an adult. Strictly speaking, one tablet is all that is necessary for either a child or an adult, but if in doubt, follow the suggestions on the container.

Remember that the recommended doses are only a guide and that with practice you will develop confidence in your own judgement.

Continuing the Dose

Several doses of a remedy may be needed before improvement occurs. The dosage scheme under the name of the chosen remedy on the right of the right-hand page will indicate the sort of timing likely to be needed. But remember that every case is different, so give the remedy more or less frequently depending on the response of the patient.

It is safe to give some remedies as frequently as every ten minutes. It is more common to give a remedy two, three or four times a day. *Whatever the circumstances, it is important that the remedy should be discontinued as soon as there is an improvement in the condition.* If you carry on for longer than is necessary you may provoke a resurgence of the original symptoms or else cause new ones to arise. (If this does happen, stop the remedy and wait for the new symptoms to subside, and then reassess the situation.)

It is difficult to be dogmatic about how long to take a remedy, since every patient is different. Usually long-term illness takes longer to treat, and short-term illness responds to treatment more quickly. But there will be exceptions. If the condition does not respond after following the dosage instructions provided, it is probable that the wrong remedy has been chosen, and it should be stopped. In this case, read the description of the symptoms again, and observe any *changes* in symptoms or *new* symptoms which may have developed in the patient. Change the remedy to suit the new symptoms.

If the original symptoms become worse, **stop taking the remedy**. This may be what homoeopaths call an 'aggravation' of symptoms and is generally a good omen. The problem is likely to get better on its own without further treatment. Later, if the same symptoms recur, take the remedy again but less often than before.

Homoeopathy is a very practical system of treatment. If the patient does not improve after using your second choice of remedy, **do not** press on regardless. The well-being of the patient is paramount, and no one should be trying to prove anything. There are occasions when other help is needed, and you should reconsider the condition of the patient. If you are in any doubt, consult a homoeopath or your own family practitioner.

Potency

The potency of a remedy is a very precise concept. It refers to the extent and the number of times the original extract of the remedy has been diluted during the preparation. As an example, Arnica 6c has been prepared as follows:

One drop of the original alcoholic extract of the Arnica plant is added to 99 drops of a solution of water and alcohol, and shaken or vibrated vigorously (in the process mentioned earlier as 'succussion'). This diluted solution is known as the first centesimal potency of Arnica, or Arnica 1c.

One drop of this new solution (1c) is diluted again in a further 99 drops of the solution of water and alcohol, shaken vigorously and so becomes the second potency (Arnica 2c).

One drop of this latest solution (2c) is added to a further 99 drops of the water and alcohol solution, vigorously shaken and this becomes the third potency (Arnica 3c).

This process of serial dilution and succussion continues through the stages to Arnica 6c. In practice any number of dilutions can be made.

It is in these repeated stages of 'potentisation' that the original substance is diluted to the point where the risk of any side-effect is eliminated. At the same time the therapeutic effectiveness of the substance is either greatly enhanced or else first becomes apparent.

The potency usually referred to in this book is 6c. It is used here because it is highly effective and also because it is the one that is most commonly available in shops in the United Kingdom.

As a rough guide, the 6c potency is used for conditions which are mainly physical, for example bruising, rheumatism or hay fever. This potency would tend to be repeated frequently, say every two hours for a day or so in the case of bruising, or three times a day for a few days for painful joints.

A more experienced prescriber may wish to give a 30c potency when the condition affects the patient more generally. The 30c potency tends to be used for illnesses which may be partly emotional in nature, such as anxiety before examinations, sleeplessness or even acute bronchitis. A few doses at intervals of every four or six hours is often all that is needed, although the effects of a nervous shock might need a few doses of a 30c every half hour or so.

Remedies in the 30c potency can be obtained either in person or by post from chemists who stock homoeopathic remedies. A current ·list of homoeopathic pharmacies is available from any of the organisations shown on page 178. There are many 'higher' potencies available in homoeopathy; that is, the remedies have been diluted and succussed many times more than the 30c potency. They should only be used by an experienced homoeopath and not by the home prescriber.

It is quite possible that you will also come across remedies in the 'x' or 'decimal' potency. These are prepared in a ratio of 1 to 9 drops instead of the 1 to 99 drops of the 'c' potency.

If you wish to prescribe a remedy but the available potency is different from the one suggested in the book, do not despair or give up. **Use the potency that you have.** It is important to remember that the fundamental reason for prescribing a particular remedy is *the similarity of the symptoms of the patient with the symptom picture of the remedy.* In principle the potency is less important than the correct choice of the remedy.

Important Points to Remember about Homoeopathic Remedies

- Remedies should be placed on the tongue and allowed to dissolve. *Do not* take with food and *do not* wash down with a drink.
- Allow about twenty minutes before or after anything else is put into the mouth. That includes foods, drinks, toothpaste, tobacco and other medicines.
- Remedies can be given in complete safety to old people, children and babies.
- They are pleasant to taste and so are popular with children.
- They are *not* poisonous – even if a child manages to swallow a bottleful (or even all the tablets in your homoeopathic medicine chest) he will come to no harm.
- They can be used in pregnancy with complete safety.
- They do not interfere with ordinary medicine, which can continue to be taken if necessary. But do not take them simultaneously. If at all possible, you should allow about twenty minutes between different medicines.
- They will be inactivated if spilled, handled more than necessary, overheated, exposed to sunlight or otherwise contaminated.
- They should be stored away from light at normal room temperatures, and away from strong-smelling substances such as scent, antiseptics, liniments or mothballs.
- The containers should be kept tightly sealed. If the remedies are kept in glass bottles they will remain active for several years. It is not known how long remedies in the new, plastic containers will remain effective. Experience suggests that it is over two years.

ACCIDENTS AND FIRST AID

ANIMAL BITES

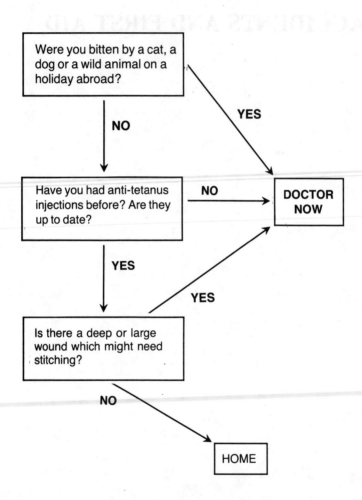

Were you bitten by a cat, a dog or a wild animal on a holiday abroad?

NO

YES

Have you had anti-tetanus injections before? Are they up to date?

NO

DOCTOR NOW

YES

YES

Is there a deep or large wound which might need stitching?

NO

HOME

ANIMAL BITES

Small bites can easily be treated at home.

By Mouth

To reduce infection and promote healing.	**Ledum 6c** and **Calendula 6c.** One dose immediately and three in the first hour. Then take one three times daily for 3–5 days.
For pain, especially in very sensitive areas, e.g. fingertips. Alternate with Calendula, if you feel that both are needed.	**Hypericum 6c.** One three times daily for 2–3 days.

Application to the Bite

Clean the wound with warm soap and water. Bathe with a freshly prepared solution of **Calendula** or **Hypercal**. This is made by adding 20 drops of the tincture to half a pint of cool, previously boiled, water. Use fresh solutions for each bathing. Dress the wound with a sterile, unmedicated dressing kept moistened with the Calendula or Hypercal solution.

BURNS AND SCALDS

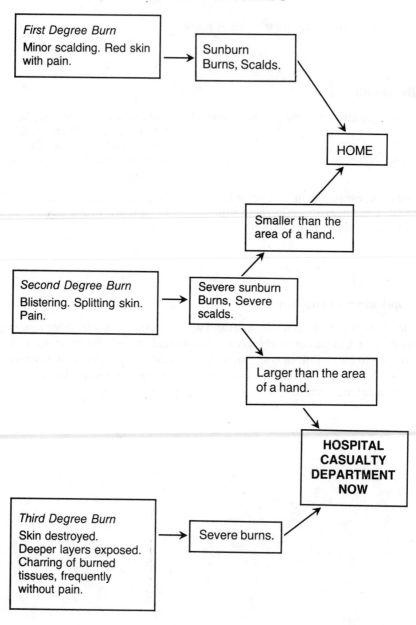

First Degree Burn

Minor scalding. Red skin with pain.

Sunburn Burns, Scalds.

HOME

Smaller than the area of a hand.

Second Degree Burn

Blistering. Splitting skin. Pain.

Severe sunburn Burns, Severe scalds.

Larger than the area of a hand.

HOSPITAL CASUALTY DEPARTMENT NOW

Third Degree Burn

Skin destroyed. Deeper layers exposed. Charring of burned tissues, frequently without pain.

Severe burns.

BURNS AND SCALDS

Immediate First Aid

Apply ice *immediately* or immerse in cold water for five to ten minutes.

Application to the Burn or Scald

Apply sterile dressings soaked in a solution of **Hypericum** or **Hypercal** or **Urtica Urens**. (The solution is made from 20 drops of tincture in half a pint of cool, previously boiled, water.)

Keep the dressing moist and disturb it as little as possible, renewing it every twelve hours or so, until the skin has healed. Apply **Calendula** ointment around the outside edge.

By Mouth

Shock and fear.	**Aconite 30c.** One dose immediately then a further three doses at fifteen-minute intervals.
Pain: First Degree with redness.	**Urtica Urens 6c.** One dose every 10 minutes or when the pain returns.
Pain: Second Degree, with cracking skin and blistering.	**Causticum 6c.** One dose every two hours until relief.
Pain: Third Degree, with destruction of deeper tissues.	**Cantharis 6c.** One dose every two hours until relief.

EYE INJURIES – BLOWS TO THE EYE

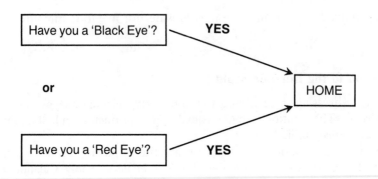

Have you a 'Black Eye'? **YES**

or

Have you a 'Red Eye'? **YES**

→ HOME

or

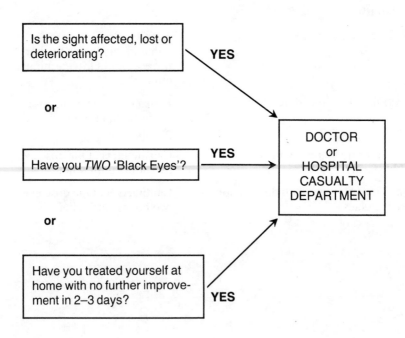

Is the sight affected, lost or deteriorating? **YES**

or

Have you *TWO* 'Black Eyes'? **YES**

or

Have you treated yourself at home with no further improvement in 2–3 days? **YES**

→ DOCTOR or HOSPITAL CASUALTY DEPARTMENT

EYE INJURIES – BLOWS TO THE EYE

Black Eye

Bruising around the eye margins with or without swelling.

Bruising (swelling) with pain.	**Arnica 6c.** One dose every two hours for 5–6 doses.
Bruising with pain. Better for cold applications.	**Ledum 6c.** One dose every two hours for 5–6 doses.
Pain in the eyeball.	**Symphytum 6c.** One dose every two hours for 5–6 doses.
Continuing pain and sensitivity externally.	**Hypericum 6c** or **Symphytum 6c.** One dose every two to three hours until the pain is reduced.

'Red Eye'

A thin layer of bright red blood in the corner of the eye.	**Hamamelis 6c.** First day one dose every 2–3 hours. Later three times daily for 2–3 days.

Conjunctivitis

Inflammation of the outer layer covering the white of the eye.	**Euphrasia eye drops in a solution.** Bathe the eye with this solution which is made up of two drops of the eye drops in an eye bath of cold (previously boiled) water.

EYE INJURIES – FOREIGN BODIES

Treat the eyes with great respect, and treat eye injuries very seriously.

Foreign Body in the Eye

Any particle, be it 'dust', stone, metal or whatever, must be removed, because of the possibility of infection and the loss of sight in that eye.

If hammering or using a power drill caused the accident, a minute particle of metal may have penetrated the eyeball.

If in doubt, visit your doctor or a casualty department immediately.

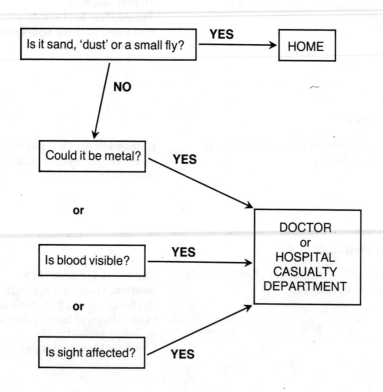

EYE INJURIES – FOREIGN BODIES

By Mouth

Shock and fear e.g. in a child.	**Aconite 30c.** One dose every half hour for 3–4 doses.
Distress and 'hysterical' anxiety, e.g. in a child.	**Ignatia 30c** or **6c.** One dose every half hour for 3–4 doses.
Pain and great sensitivity.	**Hypericum 6c.** One dose every half hour for 5–6 doses and as necessary afterwards.

Application to the Eye

Soreness may be relieved by	**Euphrasia eye drops in a solution**

Bathe the eye with this solution, which is made up of two drops of the eye drops in an eye bath of cold, previously boiled, water.

Remember, if the particle is firmly embedded, go to your doctor or to the casualty department, **without delay**.

FRACTURES

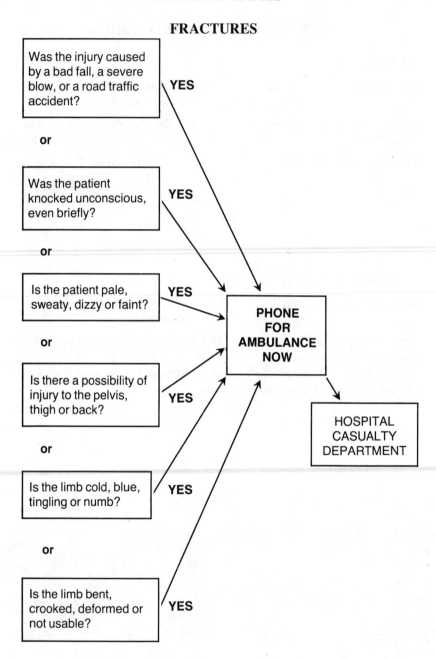

Was the injury caused by a bad fall, a severe blow, or a road traffic accident? **YES**

or

Was the patient knocked unconscious, even briefly? **YES**

or

Is the patient pale, sweaty, dizzy or faint? **YES**

or

Is there a possibility of injury to the pelvis, thigh or back? **YES**

or

Is the limb cold, blue, tingling or numb? **YES**

or

Is the limb bent, crooked, deformed or not usable? **YES**

PHONE FOR AMBULANCE NOW

HOSPITAL CASUALTY DEPARTMENT

FRACTURES

Immediate First Aid

While arrangements are made to remove the casualty to hospital.

Shock. Nervous reaction. Physical reaction – pallor, cold sweat, dizziness, nausea.	**Aconite 30c.** One dose at once and 2–3 times more if needed.
Bruising – aching pain. Injury to muscles and soft tissues.	**Arnica 6c.** One dose after Aconite and then every half hour. You may give Arnica and Aconite alternately for 2 or 3 doses.

Home Treatment after Hospital Treatment

Bruising	**Arnica 6c.** One dose twice a day until improvement.
Bone pain – along the bone or at the site of the break.	**Ruta 6c.** One dose twice daily, or
	Symphytum 6c. One dose 2–3 times daily, until relief.
Healing.	**Calc. Phos. 6c.** One a day for 1–2 months.

HEAD INJURY

Most people bang their heads at some time or another, and, beyond 'seeing stars' and suffering local tenderness and bruising, there are no other problems. So the *story* of the accident and the severity of the blow is most important in evaluating the situation.

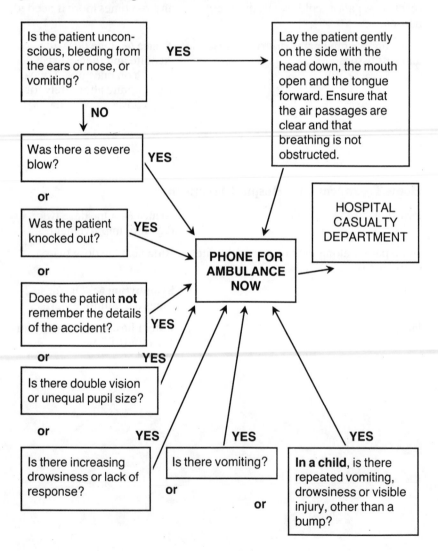

HEAD INJURY

Immediate First Aid

While the patient is being transported to the hospital casualty department or arrangements are being made, you may give the following remedies:

Shock and fear.	**Aconite 30c.** One dose immediately and repeat if the symptoms return.
Bruising. Pain. Shock.	**Arnica 6c.** One dose every half hour for 5–6 doses.
Drowsiness. Lethargy. Lack of response. Unconsciousness.	**Opium 6c.** One dose every half hour until response.

Later Treatment

Remedies commonly given after any head injury.	**Arnica 6c** or **Natrum Sulph. 6c.** One dose twice a day for 5–7 days.
Signs of brain irritation, such as spasms and muscle twitching, mental confusion and irritability	**Cicuta 6c.** One dose two to three times a day until relief or for 3–5 days.

If these symptoms suddenly occur, call your own doctor NOW.

Continuing headaches.	**Natrum Sulph. 30c.** One dose a day two to three times daily for 5–7 days.

If any symptoms persist (or return) or if you are simply unhappy with the progress of the patient, consult your own doctor.

INSECT BITES AND STINGS

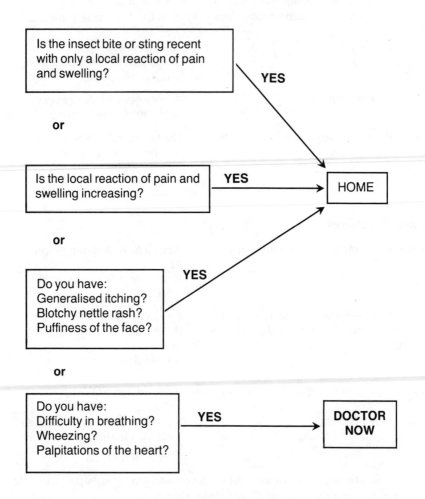

Is the insect bite or sting recent with only a local reaction of pain and swelling?

YES

or

Is the local reaction of pain and swelling increasing?

YES

HOME

or

Do you have:
Generalised itching?
Blotchy nettle rash?
Puffiness of the face?

YES

or

Do you have:
Difficulty in breathing?
Wheezing?
Palpitations of the heart?

YES

DOCTOR NOW

INSECT BITES AND STINGS

By Mouth

Shock and nervousness. Numbness and tingling. Hot, dry, burning skin.	**Aconite 30c.** One dose immediately and every half hour for 2–3 doses.
Irritation locally. Burning and stinging.	**Cantharis 6c.** One dose immediately and then every hour until soothed.
Chilly sensation, but better with *cold* applications, worse with warm applications. Worse for jarring or motion.	**Ledum 6c.** One dose every two hours for 3–5 doses.
Itchy, blotchy skin reaction; like nettle rash.	**Urtica Urens 6c.** One dose every hour until controlled.
Worse for cold, better with warmth. Irritable and sensitive to touch.	**Staphysagria 6c.** One dose every two hours until soothed.

Choose the most similar description and use that remedy. You may use two remedies alternately if you cannot make up your mind.

Application to the Bite or Sting

Bee, wasp, mosquito or midge bites and stings.	**Hypercal tincture.** Dab this on neat.

NOSEBLEEDS

Bleeding from the nose normally comes from a minor injury to the small veins in the lining of the soft part just inside the nostrils. Occasionally it occurs because of a virus infection – more frequently in children – and may start with sneezing.

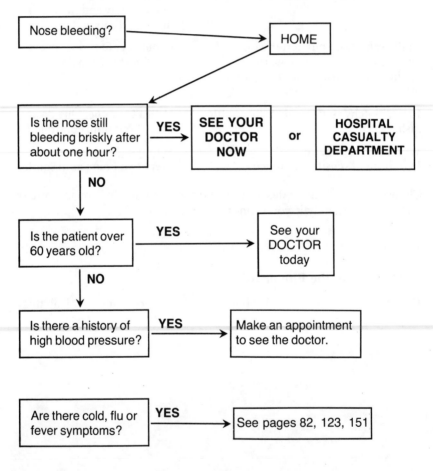

Some people have a tendency to get nosebleeds easily, and while not serious, they are a nuisance. The following method of first aid is practical, and the most suitable remedy can be given at the beginning.

NOSEBLEEDS

General Measures

- *Do not panic. Be calm.* Give the remedy.
- Sit the patient down leaning forward, over a large bowl or basin, and say 'Do not sniff or swallow the blood'.
- Use a towel as a bib to cover the chest and drape it over the knees.
- Tell the patient to *pinch* the soft part of the nose between the thumb and forefinger for *not less than five minutes by the clock*, and to breathe through the mouth throughout.
- Do not blow the nose for *twelve* hours at least.

By Mouth

After injury.

Arnica 6c. One dose every two to three hours for the first day and twice a day for 3 days.

Bright red bleeding, particularly after injury.

Phosphorus 6c. One dose every fifteen minutes until stopped.

Irritable. Fear – 'something must be done'.

Aconite 30c. One dose every half hour for 2–3 doses.

Anxious, dithery and trembly, wants to be held.

Gelsemium 6c. One dose every half hour for 2–3 doses.

Weeping. 'Hysterical'.

Ignatia 30c. One dose every half hour for 2–3 doses.

SPRAINS AND STRAINS OF JOINTS, MUSCLES AND LIGAMENTS

Joints are movable only in certain directions and the ligaments and the tissues surrounding them are easily damaged if the joint is forced into an unusual position in an accident. The ligaments may then be stretched (strain), or partly torn (sprain), or completely torn. In extreme cases the bones may be fractured or dislocated.

In all cases, sprains and strains go together with pain and swelling of the joint. The swelling lasts up to three days or so but goes down over the next ten to fourteen days. Total healing may take up to two months or more if the injuries have been severe.

Use the remedies for injuries to muscle and ligaments also, since the treatment is essentially the same.

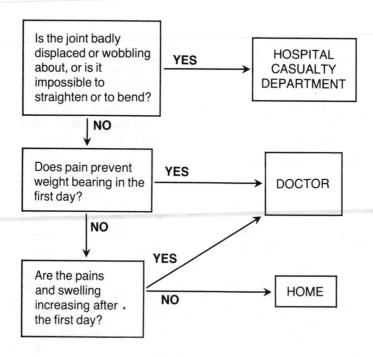

SPRAINS AND STRAINS OF JOINTS, MUSCLES AND LIGAMENTS

Immediate First Aid

While arrangements are being made to remove the casualty either to the hospital or the doctor:
- Stop all activity and weight bearing or strain.
- Reduce the swelling by applying an ice pack.
- Rest the joint in a comfortable, raised position.

By Mouth

Shock, fear or panic.

Aconite 30c. One dose every fifteen minutes for 3 doses.

Bruising and aching pain and shock.

Arnica 6c. One dose every fifteen minutes for 3 doses then one every three or four hours a day for 3–4 days.

You may take Aconite and Arnica alternatively for the first three doses.

Swelling with the skin stretched tight. *Worse for touch and pressure.* Worse for heat.

Apis Mell. 6c. One dose every two to three hours the first day and three times a day until improved.

'Bruising of bone'. Better for warmth and movement of the joint. *Worse for cold and damp.*

Ruta 6c. One dose every two to three hours the first day and three times a day until improved.

Application of Cream or Ointment to the Injury

Any of these creams or ointments can be rubbed or massaged into the skin over the injury.

Arnica. But not if the skin is broken.

Ruta or **Hamamelis** or **Rhus Tox.** These can be used if the skin is broken.

WOUNDS – ABRASIONS, SCRAPES AND GRAZES

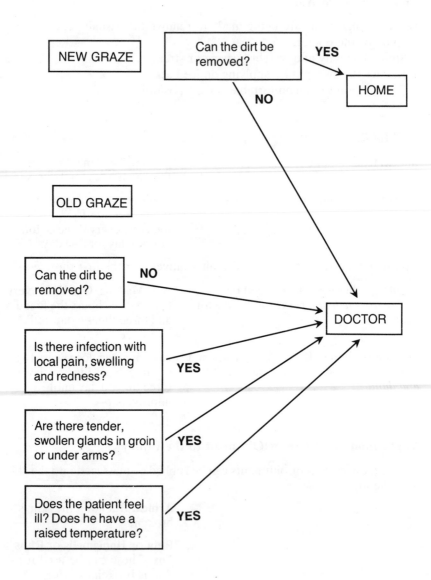

NEW GRAZE

Can the dirt be removed? — **YES** → HOME

NO → DOCTOR

OLD GRAZE

Can the dirt be removed? — **NO** → DOCTOR

Is there infection with local pain, swelling and redness? — **YES** → DOCTOR

Are there tender, swollen glands in groin or under arms? — **YES** → DOCTOR

Does the patient feel ill? Does he have a raised temperature? — **YES** → DOCTOR

WOUNDS – ABRASIONS, SCRAPES AND GRAZES

Immediate First Aid

Wash the whole area in warm, soapy water, gently scrubbing grit and dirt out with a soft brush. Rinse under the cold water tap.

Apply a dressing soaked in **Calendula** lotion. This is made by adding twenty drops of tincture to half a pint of cool, previously boiled, water.

Application to the Wound

Keep the dressing moist with the same solution (freshly made).

After two or three changes of dressings in the first day or so, disturb the dressings as little as possible. Once daily will usually be adequate.

Later, Calendula ointment may be applied when the scab has formed.

By Mouth

For possible infection and to stimulate the healing process.

Calendula 6c. One dose immediately and then four times daily for 3–5 days.

If the graze is sensitive, painful, involving areas rich in nerves (e.g. finger ends).

Hypericum 6c. One dose three times a day for 2–3 days.

Later, if there is infection with yellow pus.

Hepar Sulph. 6c. One dose three times a day for 3–4 days until clean.

WOUNDS – CUTS AND LACERATIONS

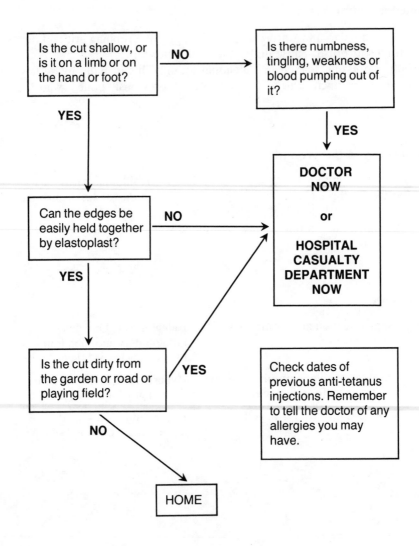

WOUNDS – CUTS AND LACERATIONS

Immediate First Aid

Wash the wound with warm, soapy water. If dirt is present, lightly scrub out the wound with a soft nail brush. Rinse under the cold tap.

Application to the Wound

Wash the cut with the freshly prepared **Calendula** or **Hypercal solution**. This is made by adding 20 drops of the tincture of Calendula or Hypercal to half a pint of cool, previously boiled, water.

Dress the wound with a sterile, unmedicated dressing kept moistened with the Calendula or Hypercal solution. Change the dressing if it becomes soaked with blood, but later only daily. If the dressing sticks to the cut, soak it off with the prepared solution.

By Mouth

Shock.	**Aconite 30c.** One dose immediately and then three further doses at fifteen-minute intervals.
Bruising. Shock.	**Arnica 6c.** One dose after the Aconite, then two or three times a day for 2–3 days.
Bleeding. Possible infection. To promote healing.	**Calendula 6c.** One dose three times a day for 4–5 days.
Pain – especially parts normally very sensitive like fingers and lips.	**Hypericum 6c.** One dose three times a day until relief.

WOUNDS – INFECTED

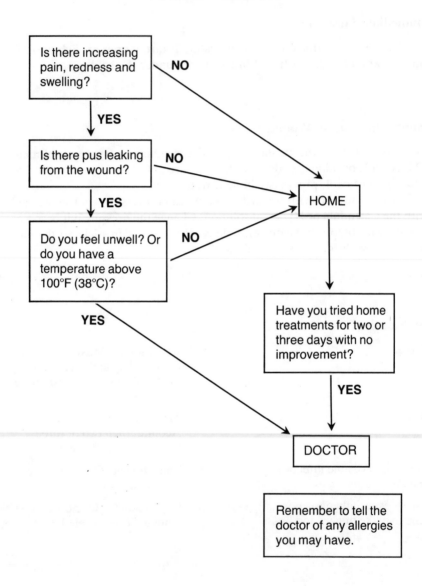

Is there increasing pain, redness and swelling?

NO → HOME

YES ↓

Is there pus leaking from the wound?

NO → HOME

YES ↓

Do you feel unwell? Or do you have a temperature above 100°F (38°C)?

NO → HOME

YES → DOCTOR

HOME ↓

Have you tried home treatments for two or three days with no improvement?

YES ↓

DOCTOR

Remember to tell the doctor of any allergies you may have.

WOUNDS – INFECTED

Immediate First Aid

Wash out the wound using small pieces of sterile gauze or clean cotton material and a freshly made solution of **Calendula** or **Hypercal**. This is made by adding 20 drops of the tincture of either of the above to half a pint of cool, previously boiled water.

Application to the Wound

Sterile dressings should be applied and kept moist with a fresh solution of either the Calendula or Hypercal. Later, Calendula ointment may be applied. Change the dressings two or three times a day to begin with. Change them less often as the pus gets less and the wound becomes cleaner.

By Mouth

To resist infection and to promote healing.	**Calendula 6c.** One dose immediately and three times a day for 3–4 days.
Pain and sensitivity.	**Hypericum 6c.** One dose three to four times a day for 2–3 days.
Wound torn and jagged, with bruising and a bruised feeling.	**Arnica 6c.** One dose three to four times a day for 3–4 days.
Infected wounds, yellow pus.	**Hepar Sulph. 6c.** One dose three to four times a day till clean.

WOUNDS – PUNCTURED

Most puncture wounds are harmless, but occasionally dirt is introduced and causes deep infection. Sometimes pieces of a sharp object may be broken off, and X-rays may be needed to locate them. In cases of infection, antibiotics and anti-tetanus injections may be required.

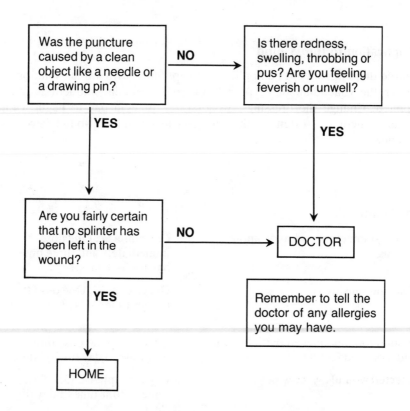

WOUNDS – PUNCTURED

Application to the Wound

Clean the wound and apply tincture of **Calendula** or tincture of **Hypercal**.

By Mouth

The basic remedy for puncture wounds is:	**Ledum 6c.** One dose immediately and three times a day for 3 days.
If a splinter remains in the wound:	**Silica 6c.** One dose four times a day until extruded.
If the wound becomes infected, i.e. throbbing pain, redness, swelling or tenderness.	**Ledum 6c.** One dose three times a day until improvement, or
	Hepar Sulph. 6c. One dose three to four times a day until improvement.

If in any doubt, consult your doctor. He may decide that tetanus toxoid injections or antibiotics are needed. Continue to use the homoeopathic remedies as well.

— NOTES —

PROBLEMS OF WOMEN

Menstruation

Menstruation is the episode of bleeding which occurs about every month during the twenty or thirty years a woman is capable of becoming pregnant. It starts in adolescence (page 40) and ends at the menopause (page 62). The loss itself consists of blood and the broken-down lining of the womb, which is shed for three to five days.

A woman may have the same menstrual pattern for years, or it may be very variable. After a pregnancy there may be a new pattern which may be permanent or temporary. The pattern may also change because of illness, physical and mental stress, or for no obvious reason.

If the pattern changes, even for no obvious reason, do not be alarmed but wait for two or three cycles to pass. Very often the cycle reverts of its own accord to the old pattern and all is well. If the old pattern is not resumed, you must consult your doctor for investigation to exclude more serious problems.

From the start of periods in adolescence most women are affected by the rhythmical rise and fall of the hormones during the menstrual cycle. Although some hardly notice anything unusual, others may complain of mental and physical symptoms. Each woman responds to these hormonal changes in her own way. Irritability, tiredness, headache, depression and pain can occur before, during and after the bleeding in any combination.

Water retention will show itself in weight gain, and more particularly, as puffiness of the face, bloating, swelling and discomfort in the abdomen and swelling and tenderness of the breasts. (See 'Premenstrual Tension', page 48).

Pain may be located in the womb, in the lower part of the abdomen, deep down in the pelvis, in the lower back, or down the thighs. (See 'Period Pains', page 46).

When a woman has period problems, she must become accurate in recording the sequence of events each menstrual cycle over three or four months, so that a typical pattern can be recognised.

The *first day* of the last menstrual bleed counts as the *first day* of the new menstrual cycle.

The following list of symptoms and when they start and finish will be found to be helpful in choosing a remedy:

- Length of the cycle (number of days from the *first day* of the last menstrual bleed to the *first day* of the new menstrual cycle.
- Length of bleeding (number of days).
- Type of bleeding – e.g. heavy, light, red, black, clots.
- Type, time and place of pains.
- Headache – especially the time in relation to the bleeding.
- Feelings – depression, weepiness, irritability, anger, tiredness.
- Weight gain – swelling of stomach, breasts, hands and feet, and the face.
- Unusual symptoms. These may be of use to an experienced homoeopath in choosing a remedy if your own choice is not helpful.

Frequently the most effective time to take the remedies is on day twelve of the cycle, although some women may find that the day after the bleeding stops is easier to remember.

One of the remedies on the right-hand page of each section may be helpful, but the picture may be complicated by emotional problems and other factors. In this case, consult other relevant pages in this section of the book and try to form a composite picture. If this fails, seek the advice of a doctor, because careful medical examination and investigation may be necessary. If these are all clear, consult an experienced homoeopath for a wider-ranging homoeopathic evaluation.

ESTABLISHMENT OF MENSTRUAL PERIODS IN
ADOLESCENT GIRLS

In Western society the age of the onset of menstruation is dropping steadily, so that even nine to ten years is increasingly common. If regular menstruation has not occurred by the middle teens, girls and their mothers become anxious. In other girls menstruation may have started normally, but later on becomes irregular, again giving rise to anxiety.

It is at this stage that the use of homoeopathic remedies is justified. However, a doctor should be consulted if their use is not successful within a few months, because he may have to examine the girl to see whether causes other than those amenable to homoeopathy may be present.

The *first day* of the last menstrual bleed counts as the *first day* of the new menstrual cycle.

A useful time to take the homoeopathic remedies for most menstrual problems is on day twelve, just two or three days before ovulation at mid-cycle.

If the last menstrual bleed was a long time before, and there is no question of the patient being pregnant, take the remedies immediately.

If it is possible that the girl is pregnant the question of re-starting the periods does not arise. The pregnancy should be confirmed by your own doctor and ante-natal care started.

ESTABLISHMENT OF MENSTRUAL PERIODS
IN ADOLESCENT GIRLS

Mild, gentle, timid. Pains, moods, mind changeable. Weeps easily, loves sympathy. Seeks attention. Jealous. Generally feels better in fresh air and for gentle exercise.

Pulsatilla 30c. Three doses, one morning, evening and the following morning, starting on day twelve of the cycle.

Irregular, variable bleeding. Premenstrual bloating. Moodiness, depression, irritability. Generally better for vigorous exercise.

Sepia 30c. Three doses, one morning, evening and the following morning, starting on day twelve of the cycle.

HEAVY PERIODS – FLOODING (MENORRHAGIA)

Heavy bleeding may or may not be painful. The fact that there is no pain *does not* mean that the underlying cause may not be serious. Tumours, fibroids, polyps, early miscarriage and hormonal imbalance must be thought of.

If heavy bleeding occurs on more than one occasion, the patient must consult her doctor. The doctor may decide that blood and smear tests would be helpful, and after an evaluation of the results in the light of the history, that a gynaecologist should be consulted.

While the patient waits for all this to happen, or when serious disease has been excluded, the use of homoeopathic remedies can very often modify or completely control the situation. The choice of the remedy should be based on the type of bleeding, the character of the pain, if present, and the more general characteristics of the patient.

HEAVY PERIODS – FLOODING (MENORRHAGIA)

Bright red bleeding on least exertion. Previous periods normal. Face and lips pale, flushing on exertion.

Ferrum Met. 6c. One dose three to four times a day during the period while still bleeding.

Heavy loss of bright red blood and clots. Changed character of bleeding, also bright red bleeding between periods. Nausea.

Ipecac. 6c. One dose three to four times a day while still bleeding.

Heavy bleeding, often late. Bearing down pains, eased by crossing legs. Low backache eased by movement.

Sepia 6c. One dose twice a day while still bleeding.

Hot, bright red blood loss. Painful cramps.

Belladonna 6c. One dose three to four times a day while still bleeding.

The remedies for this condition may also be given as three doses, one morning, evening and the following morning, starting on day twelve of the menstrual cycle. Use the 30c potency. Observe the effects over three menstrual cycles, and consult your doctor if the symptoms have not cleared up by then.

LATE PERIODS

Some women have a natural menstrual cycle which is longer than the average of twenty-eight days. This is normal for them and should not cause concern, provided that they remain well and happy.

However, some women develop delayed periods and this may make them unwell. These periods may be painful and abnormal, as a result of hormonal imbalance. This itself may arise from emotional causes, the use of the contraceptive pill, or the onset of the menopause.

Premenstrual tension occurs or increases sometimes, and this is dealt with separately (see page 48).

One of the remedies on the opposite page may be helpful, but the picture may be complicated by emotional problems, different types of pain, and feelings of malaise before, during or after the bleeding. If this is so, consult the other relevant pages in this section of the book and try to form a composite picture. If this fails, seek the advice of an experienced homoeopath.

LATE PERIODS

Thick, dark and clotted. Intermittent   **Pulsatilla 30c**
flow. Painful pressure downwards.
Gentle, yielding; highly emotional; loves
sympathy; weepy, changeable; easily
discouraged; feels better in open air.

Black, tarry blood. Flows lying down and   **Mag. Carb. 6c**
stops flowing on walking about.
Heartburn and belching.

Hot, flushing skin, rashes and spots.   **Sulphur 6c**
Faint feeling in late morning.

Blood pale. Painful colic. Generally   **Graphites 6c**
unwell and constipated. 'Morning
sickness' during period.

Late – after fright or chilling, (especially   **Aconite 30c**
in young girls whose periods are not
properly established).

Dosage. All the remedies for this condition may best be given as three doses, one morning, evening and the following morning, starting on day twelve of the menstrual cycle.

PAINFUL PERIODS (DYSMENORRHOEA)

From the start of the periods in early adolescence, most women are affected by the increase and decrease of the hormones in the blood.

Since each woman responds to the hormone changes in her own individual way, pain, irritability, headache and depression can occur before, during or after the bleeding in any combination.

The pain itself may be located in the womb, low down within the pelvis, higher in the abdomen, or in the low back. The pains may spread to the thighs.

One of the remedies on the opposite page may be helpful, but the picture may be complicated by emotional problems, different types of pain, and feelings of malaise before, during or after the bleeding. If this is so, consult the other relevant pages in this section of the book and try to form a composite picture. If this fails, seek the advice of an experienced homoeopath.

PAINFUL PERIODS (DYSMENORRHOEA)

Severe pain – sudden onset. Nervous restlessness.

Aconite 30c. One dose at fifteen minute intervals for 2–3 doses.

Cutting pain the day before period starts. Pressing down pain in right pelvis. Hot, profuse bright red bleeding. Usually better moving about.

Belladonna 6c. One dose, at fifteen to thirty minute intervals, for 3–4 doses.

Labour-like pains. Blood brown with clots. Peevish, impatient, irritable. 'Can't bear it.' 'Not fair.'

Chamomilla 6c. One dose, at fifteen to thirty minute intervals, for 3–4 doses.

Dragging down pain in left side of pelvis. Downwards pressure. Must cross legs. Bleeding early or late, scanty or profuse.

Sepia 6c. One dose, at fifteen to thirty minute intervals, for 2–4 doses.

Cutting, tearing pains in lower abdomen and back. Chilly sensation. Diarrhoea during period. Tearful.

Pulsatilla 6c. One dose, at fifteen to thirty minute intervals, for 2–4 doses.

Spasms of colic, relieved by hot water bottle. Dark, stringy blood.

Mag. Phos. 6c. One dose, at fifteen to thirty minute intervals for 4–6 doses.

Spasms of severe pain in the womb on the first day of bleeding; may seem to spread to other parts of the body. Light bleeding.

Caulophyllum 6c. One dose, at fifteen to thirty minute intervals for 4–6 doses.

The remedies for this condition may also be given as three doses, one morning, evening and the following morning, starting on day twelve of the menstrual cycle. Use the 30c potency.

PREMENSTRUAL SYNDROME (P.M.S.)
PREMENSTRUAL TENSION (P.M.T.)

Most women can recognise when a period is about to start. Some women find that for several days before a period they become unwell. These are the more common problems which occur:

- Emotional changes: irritability, depression, frustration, jealousy, 'nastiness', loss of affection for family, weeping easily for no reason.
- Fluid retention: weight gain, bloated stomach, swollen breasts, swollen hands.
- Pain: womb, deep inside pelvis, low back, thighs, headache, breasts.

In recent years women have been helped by hormone therapy, diuretics (drugs to remove retained water), and Vitamin B_6. Some women have found that Oil of Evening Primrose has been of help.

Only homoeopathic treatment, however, can actually cure the whole distressing syndrome by apparently re-establishing the correct hormone balance. Sometimes this is done within one or two menstrual cycles, and sometimes after several cycles. The patterns of symptoms to the left on the page opposite relate to four of the most commonly needed homoeopathic remedies in these situations. Their names are on the right.

Use the remedy in a 30c potency, giving one dose morning and evening and the next morning, starting on day twelve of the cycle, or at the end of a period. Use only three doses each month.

You may get a good response by finding that the expected unpleasant symptoms do not occur, or are reduced in severity. Occasionally, some symptoms (e.g. headache) may be shifted from before the period to after it. Do not be alarmed by this, but continue the treatment month by month until the symptoms have been cleared.

Then stop the remedy.

After a few symptom-free or relatively symptom-free cycles, the problems may partly return. When this occurs, *repeat the three doses for one cycle only, and wait.*

Usually the improvement tends to last for greater lengths of time and eventually only a very occasional use of the remedy is needed. Sometimes a patient may need to take the remedy in alternate cycles, or every third cycle.

If you are not able to get relief, consult an experienced homoeopath.

PREMENSTRUAL SYNDROME (P.M.S.)
PREMENSTRUAL TENSION (P.M.T.)

Breasts swollen, tender. Bearing down sensation eased by crossing legs. Womb feels as if falling out. Irregular periods. Weary, droopy, overwhelmed. Dislikes family and husband – doesn't want them. Loss of libido. Worse mid-afternoon. Better after vigorous exercise or dancing.

Sepia 30c

Bloated stomach. Swollen, tender breasts. Low abdominal pain. Moody. Negative, irritable. Selfish. Dissatisfied. Self-pitying. Blames others. Pessimistic. Takes it out on family. Hates sympathy but demands it.

Natrum Mur. 30c

Hands swollen. Clumsy and drops things. Clothes tight, needs to loosen them. Hates tight things around the neck. Spiteful, vindictive, Jealous. Unreasonable. Deliberately nasty and desires to hurt. Hates herself afterwards. Talkative. Better after bleeding starts and may pass a lot of urine then. Worse in the morning or on waking from a nap.

Lachesis 30c

Swollen breasts. Irregular periods. Thick white vaginal discharge before periods. Changeable and contradictory. Tearful. Peevish. Jealous. Loves sympathy. Over-sensitive and easily hurt. Better after gentle exercise in fresh air. Worse in stuffy atmosphere.

Pulsatilla 30c

Dosage. Read the discussion on the opposite page carefully.

SCANTY PERIODS

(A regular cycle, but the flow is short-lasting and small in quantity.)

This condition can arise in adolescence and before or during the menopause, or after pregnancy. It can also occur as part of a long illness or as a sign of general ill health, in which case consult your doctor. It may also occur after using the contraceptive pill.

If the patient remains well and happy, then do nothing. If she feels unwell in any way the use of a homoeopathic remedy may help.

One of the remedies on the page opposite may be helpful, but the picture may be complicated by emotional problems, different types of pain, and feelings of malaise before, during or after the bleeding. If this is so, consult the other relevant pages in this section of the book and try to form a composite picture. If this fails, seek the advice of a homoeopath.

SCANTY PERIODS

Pale and chilly, fat and flabby.	**Calc. Carb. 30c**
Weak, pale, gentle; moody and tearful; easily discouraged.	**Pulsatilla 30c**
Pale, thin, vivacious, but nervous and fearful. Demands constant reassurance.	**Phosphorus 30c**
Nervous, 'uptight'; holds emotions in; depression, lack of confidence. Periods may also be irregular and never · established properly.	**Natrum Mur. 30c**
Low abdominal, or bearing down pain. Constipated perhaps. Irritable, depressed; wants to be alone.	**Sepia 30c**
Caused by sudden chill or shock.	**Aconite 30c**

Dosage. All the remedies for this condition may best be given as three doses, morning, evening and the following morning, starting on day twelve of the menstrual cycle.

Problems of Women*

VAGINAL DISCHARGE (LEUCORRHOEA)

A slight discharge from the vagina is normally present in most women, and is white to pale yellow in colour. However, if it is excessive, offensive in smell, soils the underwear, or is irritating or bloodstained, medical advice must be taken.

The discharge is often, but not always, due to an infection. If there is any reason to think that it may have been caught from sexual intercourse, then the patient and the sexual partner should preferably attend the 'special clinic' at a local hospital, because of the specialised laboratory facilities they have.

In some cases medical treatment may not help, or only be helpful for a short time. **Provided that serious disease has been excluded by the appropriate medical specialists**, homoeopathic medicine may be more beneficial than orthodox medical treatments.

The remedies and dosage scheme on the page opposite will be helpful in the short term. It must be stressed, however, that for permanent benefit the patient should consult a homoeopath, who will treat the problem 'constitutionally'. Discharges of this nature often have an underlying constitutional origin, which the homoeopath is able to treat holistically, with every expectation of cure. A long-standing problem such as this may well take a long time to resolve.

Attention to hygiene and to general health is important. Avoid the use of strong antiseptics, soaps and deodorants, as sensitivity reactions may occur. Ask for 'Simple Soap' at your chemist and wash with it.

A solution of **Calendula** can be made up by adding 20 drops of the tincture of Calendula to about half a pint of cool, previously boiled water, and bathing with it.

VAGINAL DISCHARGE (LEUCORRHOEA)

Yellow, thick, ropey, sticky. Soreness, rawness, itching.	**Hydrastis 6c**
Smelly, yellow, staining. Burning pain, rawness, violent itching.	**Kreosotum 6c**
Greenish, slimy. Burning and itching. Burning urge to urinate.	**Mercurius 6c**
Smelly, brownish-yellow discharge. Itching, pricking pain in ulcers.	**Nitric Acid 6c**
Bland discharge or thick, yellowy-green; usually non-irritant but can be irritant sometimes.	**Pulsatilla 6c**
Jelly, white or yellow. Burning pain. Or dryness with discomfort when walking.	**Sepia 6c**
Thrush, continuous minor discomfort or recurring bouts of re-infection. Profuse, thick, creamy discharge. Severe itching and soreness.	**Helonias 6c**

Dosage. All the remedies for this condition may best be given as one dose morning and evening, reducing with improvement. Stop when the discharge clears. If there is no improvement consult a homoeopath.

Pregnancy

For this section the arrangement of left and right-hand pages has not been followed. Problems which may occur in pregnancy are listed with possible remedies.

Homoeopathic treatment will help greatly, but it must not in any way be regarded as a substitute for the usual ante-natal and post-natal care provided by your general practitioner and midwife.

THREATENED MISCARRIAGE

Causes Known or Suspected

Miscarriage may be caused by hormone imbalance or a fall, heavy lifting or the general overexertion and tiredness of a mother with a young family. Situations like this can threaten to destroy a pregnancy. So, particularly in women with a previous history of miscarriage or threatened miscarriage, these situations should be avoided or prevented.

The signs of a threatened miscarriage are bleeding and painful contractions. When the condition seems to develop:
- go to bed,
- rest,
- take the appropriate remedy,
- and **call the doctor**.

Hormone imbalance is frequently the cause of recurring miscarriage, especially in the early weeks of pregnancy. In this situation the patient must be cared for by an obstetrician.

A fall, followed by aching or pain in the womb with bleeding – 'a show', or 'spotting', perhaps mucus, or a loss of clear fluid.

Arnica 6c. One dose every two to four hours for about 6 doses. Use **Arnica 30c** if it is available.

Heavy lifting, resulting in dragging pain with restlessness, pressure and tenderness in pelvis, bleeding – 'a show'.	**Cinnamon 6c.** One dose every half to one hour for 4–6 doses.
Overexertion with family commitments, generally weary and tired, backache, restlessness.	**Rhus Tox. 6c.** One dose every two to four hours for 3–4 doses.

Shock

Nervous, emotional; acute hysterical reaction; weeping; extremely restless; irregular uterine pain.	**Ignatia 30c.** One dose every one to two hours for 4–6 doses.
Nervous emotional prostration; overcome by depression.	**Opium 6c.** One dose every two to four hours for 4–6 doses.
Great shock and terror; wakes with nightmares; contractions start; show of blood.	**Aconite 30c.** One dose at intervals of fifteen to thirty minutes for 2–3 doses.

'A show' or 'spotting' refers to the loss of a small amount of blood, perhaps only sufficient to soil underwear.

MORNING SICKNESS

Nausea not helped by vomiting. Usually a clean tongue; disgusted by food; irritable peevish.	**Ipecacuanha 6c.** One dose, three to four times a day, as long as needed.
Nausea – especially in the morning; especially from cooking smells; empty sensation in stomach; relieved by eating.	**Sepia 6c.** One dose three to four times a day, as long as needed.
Chilly and irritable. Belching; nausea with vomiting immediately after eating; brown coated tongue; nausea all day long without vomiting.	**Nux Vomica 6c.** One dose three to four times a day, as long as needed.

HEARTBURN

Acid burning.	**Capsicum 6c**
Acidity, worse after rich, fatty food.	**Pulsatilla 6c**
Acidity with sour taste in mouth.	**Calc. Carb. 6c**

Dosage. One dose every fifteen to thirty minutes, 4–6 times.

CRAVINGS

Pickles, sour foods and drinks; vinegar.	**Sepia 6c**
Sweets, sugar, sweet foods, fat and butter.	**Sulphur 6c**
Sweets, sugar, sweet foods, chocolate. Patient has rumbling wind.	**Lycopodium 6c**
Salty foods, extra salt. Patient has flatulence and belching.	**Carbo Veg. 6c**
Wants a variety of indigestible things; craves sour things. Moods changeable.	**Ignatia 6c**

Dosage. One dose at intervals of one to two hours, as long as is necessary.

NIGHT CRAMPS

Weary feeling in legs; cramps in calves and soles.	**Cuprum Met. 6c**
Numbness and cramps in calves and soles.	**Nux Vomica 6c**
Mind over-active; unable to sleep; tossing about; severe cramps.	**Coffea Cruda 6c**

Dosage. One dose before bed and repeat if needed.

URINARY FREQUENCY

Urging to pass urine; burning and scalding.	**Cantharis 6c.** One dose at intervals of thirty minutes to one hour and reduce with improvement.
Leaking of urine after coughing, lifting or exertion.	**Causticum 6c.** One dose three to four times daily and reduce with improvement.

See also 'Cystitis', page 130.

BACKACHE

Bruised feeling; difficulty in walking.	**Arnica 6c** or **30c.** One dose two to three times a day.
Bruised feeling. Difficulty in walking. From over-exertion.	**Arnica 6c** or **30c.** One dose two or three times a day.
Very stiff, especially after rest. Improves with continued movement.	**Rhus Tox. 6c.** One or two doses on each occasion.
Marked weakness with not too much pain.	**Phosphoric Acid 6c.** One dose two or three times a day.
Weakness and dragging feeling in small of the back. Can also be used briefly after the confinement.	**Kali Carb. 6c.** One dose two or three times a day for two or three days. Stop with improvement.

BREAST PAIN

Bryonia 6c, **Conium 6c** and **Phytolacca 6c** are all appropriate remedies for breast pain and tenderness. One dose two to four times a day. Stop with improvement.

See also 'Breastfeeding Problems', page 61, for other possible remedies.

EMOTIONAL DISTURBANCES
before (and after) confinement

Indifference to husband and children; loses interest. Depressed; bursts into tears with sympathy; 'wants to get away'. Morning sickness; nausea due to smell of cooking; loves sour drinks and vinegar.

Sepia 30c. One dose, three to four times a day, for 2–3 days.

Indifference but loves sympathy. Feels better being massaged. Afraid of being alone, the dark, thunder. Wants iced drinks; loves salt.

Phosphorus 30c. One dose a day for 2–3 days.

Moody, changeable; shy and tearful; loves sympathy. Dislikes fat, meat, butter, milk. Wants sour, refreshing drinks.

Pulsatilla 30c. One dose, three to four times a day, for 2–3 days.

'Cravings'. Craves unusual foods and is better for having them. Rapid changes of mood; contrary. Sensation of a lump in the throat. Constant sighing.

Ignatia 30c. One dose, at intervals of two to four hours, for 2–4 doses, and then three to four times a day for 2–3 days.

COMING UP TO CONFINEMENT
from eight months, i.e. 36 weeks

To Calm False Labour Pains

Sharp pains across the abdomen.

Cimicifuga 6c. One dose at intervals of half to one hour for 2–4 doses. Repeat if necessary.

To Promote Smooth Contractions of the Womb

Caulophyllum 6c. One dose a day for the last 3–4 weeks.

To Allay Anxiety and Fear

Anxiety; weakness of muscles. Trembling; 'butterflies in tummy'.	**Gelsemium 30c.** One dose and repeat as necessary.
Anxiety; sweating. 'Running to the toilet'. Hurried in everything.	**Argentum Nit. 30c.** One dose and repeat as necessary.
Anxious, restless; fastidious. Fear of death. Worse at 2 a.m.	**Arsenicum Alb. 30c.** One dose and repeat as necessary.
Anxiety tending to fear or panic. Fear of death in confinement. Palpitations. Pins and needles.	**Aconite 30c.** One dose and repeat as necessary.

COMING UP TO CONFINEMENT
last days

To reduce bruising of the tissues, and to curtail bleeding.	**Arnica 6c** or **30c.** At onset of labour pains and three times a day during and after confinement for 3–5 days.
To allay the pain and discomfort of colicky contractions of the womb.	**Caulophyllum 6c.** One dose, at intervals of one to two hours, for 2–4 doses.
To reduce the pain of 'cuts' and the injury to nerve endings.	**Hypericum 6c.** At onset of labour pains and three times a day during and after confinement for 1–2 days.

Take the Arnica and Hypericum together, as it may not be possible to remember to take them separately.

AFTER THE CONFINEMENT

Sore, bruised; bed feels hard; aches all over. Very tired.	**Arnica 6c** or **30c.** One dose as soon as possible after the birth, and three times a day for 3–5 days.
Shock; excitement; fear; sleeplessness. Unable to pass urine.	**Aconite 30c.** One dose as soon as possible and repeat thirty minutes later if necessary.
Slow labour with much stretching. Overstretched bladder. Unable to pass urine.	**Causticum 6c.** One dose and repeat thirty minutes later if necessary.
'Cuts' (episiotomy)	**Hypericum 6c.** One dose, three to four times a day, for 2–3 days.
After catheterisation, overstretching.	**Staphysagria 6c.** One dose, three times a day, for 2–3 days.

External Treatment

In order to bathe the line of stitches after being cut (episiotomy), or torn: make up a fresh solution of **Calendula** or **Hypercal** (20 drops to a half pint of previously boiled and cooled water).

Breastfeeding Problems

TOO LITTLE MILK

Milk scanty. Nursing painful, radiating to chest and neck. Mother tearful and moping. Feels worse with a hot, stuffy room. Wants fresh air.

Pulsatilla 6c. One dose, two to three times a day, and reduce with improvement.

Loss of milk. Breasts decrease in size. Thirsty and depressed.

Lac Defloratum 6c. One dose, two to three times a day, and reduce with improvement.

TOO MUCH MILK

Free flow of milk. Breasts swollen and inflamed, and very tender; red, hot and hard. Mother flushed and hot. Skin hot and dry.

Belladonna 6c. One dose every two to four hours until settled.

Free flow of watery milk. Baby refuses and cries. Breasts swollen. Patient chilly and anxious; perspires on head and face.

Calcarea Carb. 6c. One dose, three times a day, for 3–5 days and reduce.

Free flow of milk. Breasts hard and lumpy. Nipples very sore. Nursing very painful – pain radiates all over body.

Phytolacca 6c. One dose, three to four times a day, reducing with improvement.

SORE NIPPLES

Nipples inflamed; very tender; too painful to nurse. Mother irritable.

Chamomilla 6c. One dose, at intervals of thirty minutes to one hour, reducing with improvement.

Nipples cracked; very sensitive; splinter-like pains.

Acid Nitricum 6c. One dose, at intervals of one to two hours, reducing with improvement.

Pain with flow of milk; impossible to start nursing. Emotional upsets; broody and moody; ill-tempered and over-sensitive. Resentful.

Staphysagria 6c. One dose, three to four times a day, reducing with improvement.

Menopause – 'Change of Life'

The menopause occurs when the periods cease, but the problems associated with it all too frequently develop before this time and can extend beyond it.

These problems arise because of hormone imbalance. The symptoms vary greatly in their complexity and severity, as does the length of time needed by the body to create a new balance.

However, in the background of a woman's life at this time there may be emotional conflicts which arise for entirely different reasons. There may, for example, be marital disharmony, or children may be leaving the family home. Aged parents may also be causing emotional and physical stress.

It is clear that the difficulties a woman may experience at this time of her life are likely to be the complex interworking of many factors from several sources. It is unlikely that simply giving hormone replacement therapy will be enough. By the same token, it is not enough to treat the emotional problems alone. Homoeopathic remedies are especially valuable in these circumstances in that they act upon the physical and mental aspects of the individual patient.

When a woman becomes aware that she has started the change of life, it is essential that she has the benefit of a cervical smear test, internal examinaion, breast examination and so on, even if she has no symptoms that worry her.

If the medical investigations are all clear, but the remedies below have not been helpful, you should read the other sections in this part of the book to form an extended and more accurate picture. However, if none of the remedies indicated provides relief it may be the result of homoeopathic oversimplification. In these circumstances my advice is to consult an experienced homoeopath for a full evaluation.

HOT FLUSHES

Red-faced, irritable, angry, talkative, jealous, suspicious. Worse – morning and after sleep, from heat and alcohol, from tight clothes. Better – in cool air.

Lachesis 30c*

Sallow-faced, irritable, weepy, angry, depressed; loss of sexual urge; low, dragging backache. Worse – evening, extreme cold or humidity. Better – for fresh air, sleep, vigorous exercise or dancing.

Sepia 30c*

Gentle and weepy, changeable moods, needs sympathy and reassurance.
Worse – heat and humidity; tight clothes.
Better – gentle exercise and fresh air.

Pulsatilla 30c*

Hot flushes of the head and face: redness and congestion; sudden start and finish; profuse sweating of face.

Belladonna 6c. One dose at fifteen minute intervals for 3–4 doses.

Hot flushes of the head and face: as above *and* rapid palpitations of the heart.

Glonoinum 6c. One dose at fifteen minute intervals for 3–4 doses.

*Three possible dosage schemes for Lachesis, Sepia and Pulsatilla:
- One dose morning, evening and the following morning, starting on day twelve of the menstrual cycle.
- One dose morning and evening for one or two days a week.
- One dose when needed.

See overleaf for other problems associated with the menopause.

OTHER PROBLEMS ASSOCIATED WITH THE MENOPAUSE

There are other problems which can occur during the change of life. Some of these are not just menopausal and are dealt with elsewhere in this book. Some of the more particularly menopausal problems may not be 'important' from the medical point of view. However, they do make day-to-day life unpleasant and can add up to a situation affecting the woman's family and friends.

Simple measures may do away with much of the chronic low grade 'illness' of this age group. Homoeopathic remedies can be used to eliminate or reduce the need for hormones, tranquillisers, antidepressants and sleeping pills.

Arthritic pains in small joints, especially fingers. Nervous tension and anxiety, emotional instability.	**Caulophyllum 6c**
Tired, aching legs. Bruising and discolouration. Small 'burst veins'.	**Arnica 6c**
Varicose veins. Swollen, tender veins. Aching and stiffness.	**Hamamelis 6c**
Nervous and depressed. Frequent sighing, exaggerated responses, contrary emotions. Areas of numbness. Lump in the throat.	**Ignatia 30c**
Timid, sad, indecisive, emotional and weepy with music, not interested in sex.	**Graphites 30c**
Fatigue, exhaustion. Aching muscles, backache.	**Arnica 6c**

Dosage. One dose two or three times each day, reducing the frequency with improvement.

CHILDREN'S PROBLEMS

Homoeopathy is particularly helpful for the problems of children, in part because they are not generally troubled by the after-effects of repeated illnesses, or previous medical treatment, or by the build-up of chemicals from modern diets.

Remember that children fluctuate alarmingly in their symptoms in a few hours ('up one minute and down the next'), so do not panic.

Check the circumstances and the symptoms against those given in the following pages, and find the most appropriate remedy. Then give it to the child as suggested.

But remember too that babies can become more seriously unwell at a quicker rate than older children and adults. For example, a baby with diarrhoea can dehydrate rapidly in hot weather, as can a young child with an acute tonsillitis who refuses to drink because of the pain.

Homoeopathic remedies may be given to a baby as a powder. If no powders are available, the remedy in pill or tablet form may be crushed between two clean, dry teaspoons. The powder is then placed in the mouth of the baby, or dissolved in a tablespoonful of water: feed one teaspoonful per dose.

This method can be used if several doses of a remedy need to be given through the day or night.

If you have any doubts about any situation, it is essential that you consult your own doctor immediately.

The Newborn Baby

AFTER DELIVERY

Most babies are delivered quite normally without any undue problems, but occasionally the mother's labour is either prolonged or very rapid. For some reason, forceps may have to be used. In all these circumstances the baby's head will have had 'a rough passage', and homoeopathic remedies will help the bruising which may have resulted.

SOFT TISSUE SWELLING OF THE SCALP

Soft tissue swelling of the baby's scalp (caput) is normal and usually disappears in two or three days. If it persists after using Arnica and Calendula, use the other remedies, and consult your own doctor.

HERNIA

A hernia is a swelling of the local area of the wall of the tummy, frequently around the navel. Hernias protrude when the baby cries but usually they are not as serious as they look, and most disappear of their own accord.

JAUNDICE

This yellow colouration occurs in most, if not all, newborn white babies, and is quite natural. It usually becomes apparent on the second or third day after delivery and fades away two or three days after. **If the yellow discolouration deepens or continues, consult your doctor.**

AFTER DELIVERY

Particularly after a prolonged labour or a forceps delivery, or for bruising and swelling.

Arnica 6c or **30c.** Two to three doses for 2–3 days.

Calendula 6c. Two doses for 2 days, taken with the Arnica.

SOFT TISSUE SWELLING OF THE SCALP

Soft tissue swelling of the baby's scalp which persists for more than 2–3 days.

Arnica 6c. Two to three doses for 2–3 days, or

Calcarea Carb. 6c. One dose morning and evening for 3 days, or

Silica 6c. One dose morning and evening for 3 days.

HERNIA

Most hernias disappear in a few weeks. Leave them, or try:

Nux Vomica 6c. One dose twice a week for 1 month.

JAUNDICE

A mild yellowing of the skin for 2–3 days in a white baby is normal.

China 6c. One dose morning and evening for 4–5 days.

SWOLLEN BREASTS

Do nothing. This is very common, and they will go down in a few days. **Do not squeeze**.

CONJUNCTIVITIS (INFLAMMATION OF THE EYES)

This inflamed redness of the eyes occurs rarely today, because of routine use of eye drops, silver nitrate or antibiotics.

However, if it occurs and these measures are not immediately available, it is possible to use homoeopathic remedies.

Do not persist beyond two or three days before seeking further medical advice, if the baby is not making obvious improvement.

DISCHARGING EYES ('STICKY EYES')

Babies born in hospital commonly have eyes which discharge yellow pus. The cause is contamination by germs which are increasingly resistant to antibiotics. It is important to clean the eyes of the baby two or three times a day as follows:

Using a small swab of sterile cotton wool, which has been moistened with cooled, boiled water, apply gentle pressure to the inner corner of the eye and gently sweep outwards. Discard the swab and repeat the action. If necessary, use the same procedure with the other eye, using new swabs.

SWOLLEN BREASTS

If anyone has squeezed the swollen breast.	**Arnica 6c** or **30c.** Two doses a day for 2–3 days.

CONJUNCTIVITIS (INFLAMMATION OF THE EYES)

At the start, extreme redness of whites, and agitation with apparent pain and dislike of bright lights.	**Aconite 30c.** One dose and repeat as required up to three times.
Pink or red whites of eyes, (possible reaction to silver nitrate drops).	**Argentum Nit. 6c.** One dose three times a day for 3–4 days.
Pale pink, watery swelling of the whites and the lids.	**Apis Mel. 6c.** One dose every four hours for one day.

DISCHARGING EYES ('STICKY EYES')

Yellow or white discharge. Pinkness of the whites of the eyes. *Use this first.*	**Argentum Nit. 6c.** One dose every four hours for 2–3 days.
Profuse discharge of bland white or yellow pus.	**Pulsatilla 6c.** One dose every four hours for 3–4 days.
Later, 'stickiness' of the lids, especially in the morning.	**Calcarea Carb. 6c.** One dose three times a day for 3–4 days.

The Baby

FEEDING PROBLEMS

Breastfeeding is almost always best; there can be very few situations when this is not so.

The mother's milk provides the factors which defend the baby against infections before it has any immunity of its own. At the same time, the mother's milk provides the baby with the food which nature intended it to have.

There seems to be little doubt that, however carefully cows' milk is treated to make it as near as possible to maternal milk, the proteins within it remain foreign material. This may result in babies developing eczema and asthma, especially in families which have a history of allergies in general.

Milk Intolerance

This may be due to poor feeding techniques, but it may also be genuine intolerance. In this case seek advice, but do not go from one brand of powdered milk to the other needlessly.

Wind and Colic

Colic can occur without wind, and a rumbling, windy tummy need not give rise to colic. Colic is a pain tending to come and go. The baby may twist about and draw its legs up at the height of the pain.

The problem is very common, but if it continues for two or three hours, or if the baby is obviously distressed, call your doctor. A rare condition occurs when the baby suffers increasingly frequent and severe attacks of colic. It draws up its legs and cries with the pain and then falls asleep, pale and shocked-looking. The baby may then pass a loose motion with some bright red blood ('redcurrant-jelly stool'). **It is vital to call the doctor immediately or else to take the baby to hospital immediately.**

FEEDING PROBLEMS

Milk Intolerance

Great anguish; vomits everything; falls asleep after vomiting. Violent straining and thin, green, undigested stool.

Aethusa 6c. Two to three doses a day until improvement.

Chilly, fat baby with a large head. Sweats about the head; is pale and flabby; teething delayed. Chalky stools.

Calcarea Carb. 6c. Two to three doses a day until improvement.

Rejects milk, which causes diarrhoea. Swollen abdomen with loud rumbling of painful wind.

Natrum Carb. 6c. Two to three doses a day until improvement.

Wind and Colic

'Three month colic'. Whining and windy, vomiting, perhaps rejecting the milk. Pitiful crying, stops on being picked up.

Pulsatilla 6c. One dose every half hour for up to 3 doses.

Tummy blown up. Wind passed in small quantities with no relief, improved by warmth. Not much better when picked up. Irritable and obviously in pain.

Chamomilla 6c. One dose every half hour for up to 3 doses.

Chilly, irritable, angry. Overfeeding.

Nux Vomica 6c. One dose every half hour for up to 3 doses.

Writhing and twisting. Cannot keep still; better passing wind; may be caused by anger.

Colocynthis 6c. One dose every half hour for up to 3 doses.

If the condition recurs, or at any time the symptoms are severe and no relief is obtained by homoeopathic remedies, consult your doctor.

DIARRHOEA

This may be the result of bowel infection or intolerance to a particular food, if it occurs acutely. If there are recurrences, it may be due to alterations in feeding such as weaning. Teething or infections of the throat, nose or chest can also give rise to diarrhoea.

If there is an infection of any of these areas, turn to the appropriate page in the children's section and treat the condition. It is only then that the diarrhoea is likely to subside.

Remember that a baby may lose body fluids rapidly ('dehydration') and become seriously ill. This will be worse if the baby has a high temperature, is vomiting or not taking liquids or milk, or if the weather is hot. Do not hesitate to call your own doctor or take the baby to hospital if improvement does not begin in under a day.

DIARRHOEA ALTERNATING WITH CONSTIPATION

This is only likely to occur over a period of several days or even weeks, so that there is no urgency. However, attention must be paid to the general health and to the diet and liquid intake, and you should seek the advice of your doctor or the health visitor. In addition, a homoeopath may well decide to treat the baby constitutionally.

DIARRHOEA

Stools painless, very smelly and watery. Vomiting and diarrhoea together. Rapid dehydration possible. Very restless. Very thirsty.

Arsenicum Alb. 6c. One dose every two to four hours until improvement.

Pallor with white upper lip. Facial anxiety and pain. Vomiting after milk. Motion undigested, thin and green. Drowsy – not restless.

Aethusa 6c. One dose every two to four hours until improvement.

Jets of yellow, watery motion brought on by feeding.

Croton Tig. 6c. One dose every two to four hours until improvement.

Fretful baby, crying and only ceasing when held close. Legs drawn up. Slimy, watery green stool which smells like rotten eggs. Anus red and raw. Yellow stool turns green on exposure to air.

Chamomilla 6c. One dose every two hours for 4–6 doses.

Pale face, crying. Vomiting. Clean mouth and tongue. Stools putrid-smelling.

Ipecacuanha 6c. One dose every two hours for 4–6 doses.

Chilly, shivering baby. Stools copious, sour-smelling. Colicky pains and wind. Great straining with stool. May have profuse salivation and mouth ulcers.

Mercurius Sol. 6c. One dose every two hours for 4–6 doses.

DIARRHOEA ALTERNATING WITH CONSTIPATION

Perhaps with undigested food particles. Can occur in cold weather and is better in warmth.

Nux Vomica 6c. One dose three times a day for 3–5 days.

Frequently happens in warm weather.

Bryonia 6c. One dose three times a day for 3–5 days.

NAPPY RASH

This is a common skin condition, usually caused by germs in the nappy and on the skin in the nappy area. These germs break down the urine to form ammonia, which is the actual chemical cause of the rash. Detergents which are not rinsed out of nappies are also another cause.

Prevention really consists of thoroughly washing nappies and rinsing several times, with the last rinsing water containing a mild antiseptic which is dried into the nappy. An alternative practice is to use a disposable nappy.

Do *not* keep a wet or dirty nappy on the baby.

Treatment of the rash consists of allowing fresh air to get to the skin as much as conditions allow, giving the skin a chance to dry. Use bland creams or ointments before putting on the nappy. The traditional 'Zinc and Castor Oil' is generally most acceptable, but there may be individual preferences.

TEETHING

There are twenty milk teeth (baby teeth), and the first to appear at about six to ten months are the lower incisors. The last to appear are the second molars, from twenty to thirty months. A few children are born with teeth, while others do not produce the first teeth until after the first birthday. There is a very wide variation in normal children.

Most babies suffer discomfort or actual pain when teething, and produce large quantities of saliva. Gnawing and chewing on rusks or teething rings seems to give comfort. Redness around the mouth and chin will be helped by applying **Calendula** cream or ointment.

The remedies on the opposite page will help to ease the pain and general malaise. For pain with inflammation see page 148.

Other conditions such as ear infections, colds and chesty coughs occur coincidentally and are not caused by the teething. However, some babies do seem to become 'chesty' with each erupting tooth. Check the remedies for 'Cough' (page 90), and 'Colds and Influenza' (pages 82–6).

NAPPY RASH

Hot baby; red skin worse in the heat. Worse for bathing; better in the fresh air.

Sulphur 6c. One dose every day. Stop on improvement.

Chilly baby, fat and flabby. Better when warm. Sweating head at night.

Calcarea Carb. 6c. One dose three times a day. Stop on improvement.

TEETHING

Chilly, fat and flabby. Sweating head at night.

Calcarea Carb. 6c. One dose three times a day. Stop on improvement.

Chilly, but thinner and wiry.

Calcarea Phos. 6c. One dose three times a day as required.

Very painful. Intense irritability. Can't be settled down. Angry, and helped by carrying. Diarrhoea – green, offensive smell.

Chamomilla 6c. One dose and repeat if necessary.

THE CRYING BABY

The first thing to do is to check what is wrong or, indeed, if anything is wrong at all:
- Is there a fever?
- Does the baby look ill?
- Does the nappy need changing?
- Has the baby passed a motion? Is it loose and offensive?
- Does the baby need feeding?

See other pages in this section for conditions such as teething, colic, diarrhoea, etc.

CONVULSIONS (FITS)

The baby usually has an infection with a high temperature which affects the working of the brain. The fit normally shows itself as a twitching of the face, arms and legs and occasionally the whole body. The breath is held and the skin becomes deep red and then a blotchy purple. After a few seconds the twitching stops, the breathing restarts and the baby becomes pink again.

All of this is alarming to the parents, but usually fits look worse than they are.

The first steps are:
1) Remain calm.
2) Unclothe the baby.
3) Cool it down by bathing it in warm water.
4) At the same time give the remedy indicated.

If the baby does not settle down or if further fits occur, **call the doctor now**. If the condition settles, consult the doctor at the first suitable time.

THE CRYING BABY

Whimpering, 'whingeing', stops when cuddled. Wants affection.	**Pulsatilla 6c.** One dose and repeat if necessary at fifteen minute intervals for up to 4 doses.
Whining and rejecting. Doesn't want to be picked up. Worse for touching.	**Antimonium Crud. 6c.** One dose and repeat if necessary at fifteen minute intervals for up to 4 doses.
Angry, over-sensitive. Chilly; better for warmth.	**Nux Vomica 6c.** One dose and repeat if necessary at fifteen minute intervals for up to 4 doses.
Angry, excitable, irritable, lashes out. Inconsolable; not helped by picking up.	**Chamomilla 6c.** One dose and repeat if necessary at fifteen minute intervals for up to 4 doses.

CONVULSIONS (FITS)

Hot, red with fever. Dilated pupils.	**Belladonna 6c.** One dose and repeat in fifteen minutes if necessary. Continue every two to three hours for 1–2 days, to treat the underlying infection.
Teething. Extremely agitated; violently restless.	**Chamomilla 6c.** One dose and repeat in fifteen minutes if necessary.
Anger and irritation.	**Nux Vomica 6c.** One dose and repeat in fifteen minutes if necessary.
After fright.	**Ignatia 6c.** One dose and repeat in fifteen minutes if necessary.

Toddlers and School Children

ADENOIDS – LARGE

(Nasal voice, mouth breathing, snoring, dull hearing or intermittent deafness.)

This condition frequently occurs with a cold, and sometimes with acute tonsilitis. Usually when the immediate illness subsides, so do the adenoids; but not always. In this case a long-term problem arises.

Remember that it may be necessary for the child's well-being to use antibiotics in certain circumstances, and their use should not be spurned out of hand. However, repeated doses of antibiotics are not helpful. Antihistamines and drying agents also give rise to many problems. They may help in the short term, but if used at all should only be used very sparingly.

While it is true that this situation settles down by about the age of 10 or 11 years, an awful lot of trouble can arise before then. The general poor health and unhappiness and the loss of school time worries parents.

The use of homoeopathic remedies in the sudden, acute stages can be very helpful.

Another way of using remedies is to 'build up the resistance' of the child. This is probably best done after thoughtful enquiry into the family background by a homoeopath.

FLUID IN THE EARS ('GLUE EAR')

This usually occurs after ear infections following a cold. It may only last a few days, but it may take many weeks to clear. Your doctor should be consulted if deafness or poor hearing persists, in order that the level of hearing can be monitored.

If ear, nose and throat infections are promptly and correctly treated, 'glue ear' is not likely to occur. However, if the condition has been present for a long time, treatment using only 'first aid' homoeopathic remedies is unlikely to be enough. In this situation, it would be wise to seek the advice of an experienced homoeopath, who will evaluate the whole person, taking into account the patient's past history and the family history.

ADENOIDS – LARGE

Green-yellow catarrh. Mouth breathing. Squelching in the ears with dull hearing. Whining and wants to be cuddled. Can be better in fresh air.

Pulsatilla 6c. One dose twice a day for 10–14 days.

Snuffling, snoring. Glands in throat and neck swollen. Swallowing difficult. Feels the cold, catches cold easily.

Silica 6c. One dose twice a day for 10–14 days.

Constant mouth breathing. Tonsils and neck glands enlarged. Poorly developing child both mentally and physically.

Baryta Carb. 6c. One dose twice a day for 10–14 days.

All these short courses of treatment may have to be repeated if the symptoms return.

FLUID IN THE EARS ('GLUE EAR')

Deafness – intermittently hard of hearing. Variable deafness. Squelching, bubbling noises in the ear.

Pulsatilla 6c. One dose morning and evening for 4–8 weeks. Or **Kali Mur. 6c.** One dose morning and evening for 4–8 weeks.

If the treatment appears to cure the deafness, and your doctor finds on examination that the ear drums have returned to normal, then stop.

If however the ear drums have not completely returned to normal, or the hearing is improving but variable, continue to use the remedies for a further month and arrange for your doctor to examine the ears again.

If there is still doubt, ask to be able to consult an E.N.T. surgeon.

BEDWETTING

Bedwetting occurs when the control of the bladder is lost during sleep and urine is passed unconsciously. Some children may never have developed bladder control at night.

Other children may be incontinent during the day also. This may be due to 'being lazy' – they may be far more interested in what they are doing, and rush to the toilet too late. Usually it is best to train the child to use the toilet at fairly regular intervals.

A far smaller group of children may leak fairly constantly all day and all night. These children need to be taken to the family doctor for possible investigation into the anatomy and nervous control of the bladder.

By far the largest group of children simply 'wet the bed'. If the child is sensitive and anxious, the cause may be obvious and the treatment is to support and to encourage the sufferer. This will reduce the bed-wedding and the source of anxiety.

General Management

- Sympathy and encouragement, and a praise instead of blame approach is best. Ignore wet nights but give 'stars' for the dry nights.
- The incontinence pad with an alarm bell may help the deep sleepers, and can be arranged by your own doctor and health visitor.
- Avoid giving the child large drinks in the late evening and before going to bed.
- Arrange for the child to use the toilet three times before bed time, say half an hour, a quarter of an hour and immediately before getting into bed.
- Arrange for either parent to 'lift' the child when they go to bed themselves.

Whilst doing all or any of these things, use homoeopathic remedies as an aid. However, for many of these children bedwetting may be a problem of long duration. If these remedies are not helpful, seek the advice of an experienced homoeopath.

BEDWETTING

Large quantities of urine. 'Soaks the bed' early in sleep.

Plantago 6c. One dose each night for 5–10 days.

'Soaks the bed' later in sleep. Anxious and irritable.

Lycopodium 6c. One dose each night for 5–10 days.

Wet during the day also. Leaks with coughing. Wet in early sleep; not aware of passing urine.

Causticum 6c. One dose three times a day for 5–10 days.

'Soaks the bed'. Dreams and nightmares. Discomfort and tenderness in the bladder. (Consult the doctor about possible infection.)

Equisetum 6c. One dose six times a day for 5–10 days.

Wet in first sleep.

Sepia 6c. One dose three times a day for 5–10 days.

COLDS AND INFLUENZA

Not much can be done to prevent children from being exposed to viral infections at school. Indeed, their first years at school are frequently a long succession of infections.

If the child is basically healthy there is little to worry about, since children benefit from developing immunities to all the germs they encounter. Each illness can be satisfactorily dealt with using homoeopathic remedies, as indicated by the patient's symptoms, and each illness can be regarded as a necessary stepping stone to maturity.

The problem arises when the child goes from one illness to the next without ever recovering properly. They can be made to feel even worse by the prescription of antibiotics. In this situation the use of 'Cold and Influenza tablets' (made up by the major homoeopathic manufacturers) taken at monthly intervals around the year, can be very effective in reversing the trend.

Prevention

A good diet is essential, with a plentiful supply of fresh fruit and vegetables.

Additional vitamins, especially vitamin C during and after illness should be taken in the quantities recommended by the particular manufacturer. Many people believe that extra vitamin C prevent infections. It may do so, and the fact that medical scientists have not proved the matter one way or the other need not prevent you from playing safe.

Children need plenty of exercise, and should take enough to become healthily tired. They should be in the open air as much as possible, exposed to sunshine, care being taken to avoid over-exposure and sunburn.

COLDS AND INFLUENZA

Prevention

> **'Cold and Flu tablets'.** One dose morning and evening on the first day of each month through the year, and perhaps every two weeks during the winter.

This method of prevention should be continued only until the child has obviously improved in general health, and has not had bad colds, sore throats, catarrh and ear problems during the previous winter. If they have been successfully treated, a cold will have been short-lived and recovery complete.

COLDS AND INFLUENZA

Treatment – First Signs – First Stages

- Use the homoeopathic remedies as indicated by the main symptoms of the patient, changing them as the picture changes, if necessary.
- Rest the child, preferably in bed, but downstairs if it will not settle easily. The room should be light and airy; the patient should not be over-clothed and allowed to become too hot.
- The child should be encouraged to drink as much as possible.
- Remember that as the child recovers, it will need toys and games and puzzles to occupy its mind. Try to avoid the hypnotic effect of too much television.

COLDS AND INFLUENZA

Treatment – First Signs – First Stages

Starts in frosty weather and very cold, dry winds. Restless, feverish, shivering. Coldness. Sneezing, dry cough. Tickling in the throat.

Aconite 30c. One dose every 1–2 hours until improvement.

Starts in cold weather and very cold dry winds. Stuffed-up, dry nose. Very shivery, cold and irritable. Sore throat, backache. Unable to get warmed.

Nux Vomica 6c. One dose every 1–2 hours until improvement.

Chilly, restless, weakness. Watering eyes. Burning sensation in a running nose, sneezing with no relief. Thirst for cold drinks.

Arsenicum Alb. 6c. One dose every 1–2 hours until improvement.

Frequent sneezing bouts. Watery nose – irritates upper lip and nose. Watery eyes – painless.

Allium Cepa 6c. One dose every hour until improvement.

Slow onset in mild, damp weather. Dullness, heavy-eyed look. Ache in head, neck and shoulders spreading to arms and legs. Weakness, mild fever. Lump in the throat.

Gelsemium 6c. One dose every 1–2 hours until improvement.

Chilly after getting wet. Worse in damp conditions or damp weather. Sneezing and stuffiness.

Dulcamara 6c. One dose every 1–2 hours until improvement.

Bouts of sneezing. Irritating tears and red-rimmed eyes. Running nose – not irritant.

Euphrasia 6c. One dose every 1–2 hours until improvement.

COLDS AND INFLUENZA

Treatment – Later Stages

There is a more or less gradual resolution of the illness, from a clear, watery mucus to a thick and coloured catarrh. The general care of the patient is not likely to change very much, but the symptoms may do so. If they do, care must be taken to change the homoeopathic remedy.

Some remedies representing the later stages of a cold are on the opposite page. By using them you will find that the infections will tend to be shorter and less troublesome, with a quicker restoration of good health.

Chesty Cold

In some patients a cold always 'goes on to the chest'. There is often a family tendency to respond in this way. While the remedies given opposite may be helpful each time, only constitutional treatment by an experienced homoeopath is likely to eradicate the tendency.

COLDS AND INFLUENZA

Treatment – Later Stages

Sneezing with a sore, running nose. Sore upper lip. Red watery eyes. Worse indoors, better for fresh air.

Allium Cepa 6c. One dose every two to three hours until improvement.

Cold starts in nose, travels to chest. Sore throat. Hard, dry, painful cough. Irritable; splitting headache.

Bryonia 6c. One dose every two to three hours until improvement.

Thick, greeny-yellow catarrh. Stuffy nose at night and indoors. Runny nose in morning and outdoors. Generally feels better in fresh air.

Pulsatilla 6c. One dose every two to three hours until improvement.

Cold spreads to throat. Bad breath. Restless with throbbing, tight headache. Chilly and trembling. Greenish nasal catarrh. Chesty cough.

Mercurius Sol. 6c. One dose every two to three hours until improvement.

Weakness, stiffness, soreness of muscles. Severe aching deep in bones and eyes. Fever.

Eupatorium Perf. 6c. One dose every two to three hours until improvement.

Chesty Cold

Onset of chest infection. Painful, dry or moist cough. Fever, pulse rapid.

Ferrum Phos. 6c. One dose every two to three hours until improvement.

Wheezy bronchitis, phlegm on chest. Breathing noisy and difficult. Nostrils dilated and moving in and out with breathing.

Antimonium Tart. 6c. One dose every two to three hours until improvement.

Stabbing pain. Dry, spasmodic cough, made worse by slightest movement, coughing or sneezing.

Bryonia 6c. One dose every two to three hours until improvement.

CONSTIPATION

General Management

- Encourage the child to use the toilet at regular times, but do not cause resentment or anxiety in the process.
- Train the child to go to the toilet as soon as the urge to empty the bowels occurs. This is easier said than done, especially when the child is reading, playing or watching TV.
- Drinking adequate quantities of water will help to prevent the motions from becoming hard. Remember that the child will require more drinks in very hot weather, or if it is unwell with a high temperature.
- Increase the amount of 'roughage' in the diet. This is best done by giving wholemeal bread and cereals, and by increasing the quantity of fruit and vegetables eaten daily. At the same time eliminate the highly refined and manufactured foods. In short – cut out 'junk food' and provide a 'wholefood' diet.

CONSTIPATION

Straining for a soft sticky stool. Unable to pass stool until a large accumulation. Older children who eat indigestible things.

Alumina 6c. One dose two to three times a day and reduce with improvement.

Frequent and ineffectual desire. Small quantities at each attempt. Alternating with diarrhoea. Impatient and over-sensitive.

Nux Vomica 6c. One dose morning and evening, reducing with improvement.

No desire for stool. No complaints. Bowels seem closed.

Opium 6c. One dose morning and evening, reducing with improvement.

COUGH

Coughing is a symptom of irritation in the air passages. It can flare up suddenly with the breathing in of dust, smoke or fumes. However, with children, coughs are most likely to occur because of colds and throat or chest infections.

For the convenience of prescribing homoeopathic remedies, coughs can be divided into three groups, although there is likely to be an overlapping of symptoms:

- *Dry cough* – e.g. laryngitis.
  This cough is harsh, short and painful.
- *Spasmodic cough* – e.g. whooping cough.
  This cough is repetitive and may have a tight wheeze in the chest. Children tend to retch or even vomit at the end.
- *Loose cough* – e.g. a 'chesty cold'.
  This cough produces varying amounts of phlegm or sputum. If the phlegm is thick, sticky and coloured green or dusky-red, you should consult your own doctor who may need to prescribe an antibiotic.

General Measures

It is usually wise to keep the patient indoors in a warm, airy room if the weather is bad, and to avoid changes in temperature or places where the cough is worsened, in order to prevent fresh outbursts of coughing.

Check the symptoms of the patient and choose the most suitable remedy on the page opposite.

If the child has a cold or virus infection, it may also help to refer to the sections on colds and influenza and croup (see pages 82–7 and 92) and try to form a composite picture. You may give a remedy on its own; but if you cannot decide which of two is the better, give them alternately.

Call the doctor if:
- The overall condition worsens.
- The child has other medical problems.
- Progress is not being made in a reasonable time – say three or four days.

Sometimes coughs can drag on for weeks. In other cases, the child may have repeated infections over a period of years. In both these situations the child can be said to have a basic weakness, and this can only be treated on constitutional grounds. Such treatment is beyond the scope of this book and you should consult an experienced homoeopath.

COUGH

Dry Cough

Croup-like cough in very dry, cold weather. Anxiety and restlessness. Fever, thirst, no sweating.

Aconite 30c. One dose every fifteen minutes, reducing with improvement.

Rough, noisy croup-like cough. Sudden onset in cold weather. Better in a warm, steamy room.

Hepar Sulph. 6c. One dose every fifteen minutes, reducing with improvement.

Raw, tearing, burning pain in a croup-like cough. Improves with hot drinks.

Spongia 6c. One dose every fifteen minutes, reducing with improvement.

Slow gradual fever; irritation of air passages. Cough worse for movement and entering a warm room; can be worse at night. Much thirst for cold drinks. Stabbing pains in throat or chest.

Bryonia 6c. One dose every fifteen minutes, reducing with improvement.

Spasmodic Cough

Bouts of dry cough – a bit like whooping cough. Worse at night and lying down. May be wheezing; occasionally croup-like.

Drosera 6c. One dose, repeated when necessary, or one dose at intervals of 4–6 hours.

Crowing spasmodic cough. Better sipping cold water.

Cuprum Met. 6c. One dose every fifteen minutes until improvement.

Spasms of coughing. The more he coughs, the more he has to.

Ignatia 6c. One dose morning and evening and after a bout of coughing.

Loose Cough

Spasmodic cough, worse in open air. Breathless. Rapid development of phlegm which may be vomited up.

Ipecacuanha 6c. One dose every hour until improvement.

Thick yellow loose phlegm. Runny nose. Cough productive in day and dry at night, better in fresh air. Towards end of illness.

Pulsatilla 6c. One dose three to four times a day.

Loose phlegm, thick and difficult to cough up. Breathless. Wheezing, noisy chest.

Antimonium Tart. 6c. One dose four to six times a day.

CROUP

This is a spasm of the vocal cords which makes *breathing-in* difficult, giving a sensation of suffocation. It usually occurs at night. The child may already have a cough or a cold, but it can come 'out of the blue'. It causes a crowing or croaking noise, frequently with a barking or metallic cough.

All this makes the child and the parents frightened, which again aggravates the problem, creating a vicious circle of spasm, breathing difficulty, and fear.

The attack may last from one to three hours and then rapidly ease off, but it can recur for two or three nights.

Croup can be dangerous and should not be ignored.

Treatment – General Measures

- Be **calm** and **soothing** and **reassuring**.
- Handle the child gently. Sitting up is usually the best position but cuddle the child in its favourite position.
- Use the homoeopathic remedies listed on the opposite page.
- Create a warm moist atmosphere in the room, using a steadily steaming kettle to help with this.
- **Call your doctor** if there are no obvious signs of improvement in 30–60 minutes, or if at any time the spasm worsens or the breathing becomes difficult, or if the colour of the lips and fingernails of the child turn blue.

CROUP

Take in order:

Use at the early stage of any fever but especially to allay fear. Use first in croup.	**Aconite 30c.**
Can also be helpful in suffocating coughing spells. Worse in cold atmosphere. Worse with cold draughts.	**Hepar Sulph. 30c or 6c.**
Can also be helpful for the child who wakes from sleep, choking with a violent cough.	**Spongia 30c or 6c.**

The recognised treatment for croup is first to give a dose of Aconite 30c, followed in ten to fifteen minutes by Hepar Sulph. and by Spongia ten to fifteen minutes after that. Then return to the Hepar Sulph., continuing the treatment as required by alternating Hepar Sulph. with Spongia at ten to fifteen minute intervals. Use whatever potency is available, but the 30c is likely to be more powerful.

Note the condition of the child. **Call the doctor if there is no easing of the croup or if it gets worse.**

EARACHE

This is usually caused by infection behind the eardrum, having developed from infection of the throat and nasal passages. The eardrum becomes inflamed and painful. Pus forms behind the eardrum, increasing the pressure and forcing the drum to bulge outwards. This increases the pain. At the same time the child becomes very unwell and 'toxic' with a fever.

If homoeopathic remedies appropriate to the particular child are used quickly, the whole sequence may be stopped, and the child will recover quickly.

Remember, middle ear infection is a potentially dangerous condition which should not be neglected. A doctor should be consulted if the child does not appear to respond to treatment quickly. It may be necessary to use antibiotics as well as homoeopathic remedies.

If the above situation is a one-off event and the treatment suggested is successful, then that is the end of the matter. But if the earache is repeated several times each winter, or forms part of a picture of frequent colds and chest infections, there is an underlying constitutional weakness which can only be helped by 'constitutional' treatment. You must consult an experienced homoeopath for this.

EARACHE

Abrupt onset of pain in ear, especially after a chill in cold, dry weather. Unbearable and usually worse at night, some improvement by local heat, skin burning and dry; fever with shivering. Anxious and restless, fearful.

Aconite 30c. One dose at intervals of thirty minutes for 3–4 doses.

Throbbing pain, not so rapid onset. Very hot dry skin, red face and dilated pupils. Not restless or fearful.

Belladonna 6c. One dose at intervals of thirty minutes and reduce with improvement.

Jerking, tearing pain, ears hot. Pain is made worse by heat. Miserable and whining; responds to cuddling and affection.

Pulsatilla 6c. One dose at intervals of thirty minutes and reduce with improvement.

Stabbing pain, intolerable. Cross, irritable; doesn't know where to put himself.

Chamomilla 6c. One dose at fifteen to thirty minute intervals and reduce with improvement.

Pain, stinging, burning, pricking. External ear may be red and tender. Eased by cold compresses; made worse by heat. Hot dry skin alternating with perspiration.

Apis Mell. 6c. One dose at intervals of thirty minutes and reduce with improvement.

EARS – DISCHARGING

Discharge may arise from the walls of the canal leading down from the outer ear to the eardrum. But it is safer to remember that it can arise from the bursting of the eardrum by the pressure of pus behind it.

Earache which ceases suddenly followed by the appearance of pus discharging from the ear canal probably means that the eardrum has burst. This is not an emergency because the pressure in the ear has been relieved – when the infection has subsided with treatment the eardrum will heal. The perforation will close and hearing will return to normal.

Use homoeopathic remedies which may already be helping, or change to a remedy which is indicated by the type of pus being discharged.

For ears which have discharged many times – 'chronic ears' – it would be better to consult an experienced homoeopath.

It may be necessary to use antibiotics. If this course is decided upon, it will be helpful to use homoeopathic remedies at the same time.

EARS – DISCHARGING

Yellow pus – flows easily. Very sensitive to draughts.	**Hepar Sulph. 6c.** One dose three times a day until improvement.
Yellow-green pus; thicker, sticky.	**Pulsatilla 6c.** One dose three times a day until improvement.
Thick, white, stringy pus; very sticky and difficult to clean.	**Kali Mur. 6c.** One dose three times a day until improvement.
Foul-smelling pus.	**Pyrogenium 6c.** One dose three times a day until improvement.

When the discharge stops, continue the original treatment for two further days, and then give **Sulphur 6c** morning and evening for two days more.

FEVERS AND INFECTIOUS DISEASES IN GENERAL

Epidemics

Thanks to a combination of several factors, including better nutrition and housing, better control of water supplies and sewerage disposal, and perhaps routine immunisation measures, some infectious diseases have ceased to be of major importance in Western society.

Immunisation

Unfortunately, whilst immunisation has been of great benefit in controlling infections like diphtheria, tetanus and poliomyelitis, some children have suffered severe reactions. Of these children a very small number have been permanently damaged.

All parents must decide about the use of vaccines for their own children. After taking advice from the doctor, the responsibility is theirs.

Children who have any of the following should either be immunised with great caution or not at all:

- Convulsions or a family history of convulsions or epilepsy.
- A bad reaction to previous immunisation.
- A family history of asthma or wheezing.
- A family history of allergies of any sort.
- A family history of infantile eczema.

Homoeopathic remedies made from disease products (nosodes) are useful as an alternative. Although they have been used for many years and have no side effects or reactions, the degree of protection they provide has not yet been scientifically established.

General Management

- Dress in light clothes in a warm, well-ventilated room,
  – or –
- Put to bed with light clothing.
- Do not overwrap or cover up the patient, or in any way raise the temperature to 'sweat it out'.
- If the temperature is raised, cool the child down by bathing it or allowing it to play with toys in the bath for longer than usual.
- Provide *and give* frequent drinks.

FEVERS AND INFECTIOUS DISEASES IN GENERAL

First signs of onset: Dry, burning skin. **Aconite 30c**
Fever. Thirst, chills. Restlessness and
anxiety. Worse in evening and before
midnight.

Early stage with high fever: Dry, burning **Belladonna 6c**
skin. Red face. Dilated pupils. Swollen,
tender glands.

Restless and agitated. Great anxiety. **Arsenicum Alb. 6c**
Prostration. Needs warmth except to
head. Hot and cold alternately. Thirsty
for small amounts. Worse after midnight.

Very drowsy and confused. Dull-looking. **Baptisia 6c**
Hallucinations. Temperature irregular.
General bruised sensation.

Shivery and sweating. Thirsty for large **Bryonia 6c**
amounts at long intervals. Headache and
pain. Worse for jarring and coughing.

Heavy aching feeling of limbs and head. **Gelsemium 6c**
Drowsy. Slow onset, trembling. No
thirst. Chills up and down spine.

Low grade fever – slow onset. Moderate **Ferrum Phos. 6c**
thirst. Frequent sweats. Shivering,
headache. Generally not much to show
for the condition as a whole.

Remember that a few doses of Aconite 30c at intervals of about an hour, started at the very first signs of an illness, can hasten its resolution and even abort it.

However, if the above symptoms are established give the appropriate remedy as follows: One dose every one to two hours for the first day, and reduce the frequency with improvement over the next two or three days.

MEASLES

After starting like a common cold, the dull blotchy red rash starts behind the ears and spreads to the face, trunk and limbs. The face is puffy and the eyelids swollen. Dislike of strong light is helped by drawing curtains and using heavily shaded lights. Light will *not harm* the eyes, only cause discomfort.

CHICKENPOX

In young children small pink spots start on the back and spread to other parts. They become fluid-filled vesicles like small glass beads or drops of water *on* the skin. Later they become yellow. The main problem is intense itching caused by the vesicles. Calamine lotion dabbed onto the skin can be very soothing. Treatment can be of the general condition and of the skin irritation.

MEASLES

Prevention and contact: children not immunised and other children in the family.

Morbillinum 30c or **Pulsatilla 30c.** Three doses in 24 hours.

Early Stages: (see 'Fevers', page 99).

Later Stages
Restless, whingeing, wants petting and comforting. Cough troublesome. Wants cool air.

Pulsatilla 6c. One dose three to four times a day for 4–5 days.

Chesty – tight feeling, dry cough. Very thirsty, wants cold water which he may vomit.

Phosphorus 6c. One dose three to four times a day for 4–5 days.

High temperature; chilly shivers. Dull look, swollen face, chesty. Cough causing headache.

Bryonia 6c. One dose three to four times a day for 4–5 days.

Running nose; watering, sore eyes. Strong light painful. Not very ill.

Euphrasia 6c. One dose three to four times a day for 4–5 days.

CHICKENPOX

Prevention and contact: with friends with chickenpox.

Rhus Tox. 30c. Three doses in 24 hours.

Pustules large. Peevish and whining. Wants company.

Antimonium Tart. 6c. One dose three to four times a day for 4–5 days.

Peevish, cries easily. Hates being touched or washed.

Antimonium Crudum 6c. One dose three to four times a day for 4–5 days.

Restless mind and body. Great itching.

Rhus Tox. 6c. One dose three to four times a day for 4–5 days.

Continue using the remedy for two or three days after the main symptoms clear up. Ask your doctor's advice if you have any doubts about new symptoms or any worsening of the condition.

WHOOPING COUGH
(See also 'Cough', page 90)

This can be dangerous under the age of six months, and very troublesome under the age of one year. Starting like a cold, the harsh, dry coughs become grouped together and finally a whoop develops, with prostration and vomiting. (See note on page 98 about immunisation.) In any event, Pertussin may be used in an attempt to prevent whooping cough and as an aid to recovery afterwards.

SCARLET FEVER

This illness begins with headache, sore throat, painful neck glands and a high fever. The fine flush of a rash begins on the second day except around the mouth. This disease practically disappeared from the scene in the United Kingdom for about twenty years, but has returned with an increasing frequency in the last ten years or so. The problem here is the possibility of developing complications in the heart and kidneys, and because of this it is essential to consult your doctor at the outset. Remember to warn the doctor about any possible allergy to antibiotics.

Homoeopathic remedies are valuable when used together with your doctor's orthodox treatment. You may use the first-aid remedies on the page opposite, **but only to give you time to arrange to consult an experienced homoeopath.**

WHOOPING COUGH
(See also 'Cough', page 90)

Prevention and contact during outbreaks in your district.

Pertussin 30c. One dose once a week for the duration of the outbreak (on prescription only).

Very Early Stage

Dry, hard, ringing cough. Fever, thirst, hot skin. Rapid pulse. Anxiety.

Aconite 30c. One dose every two hours for 2–3 doses.

Barking, repetitive cough. Worse at night. Restless, crying. Hot, red, dry skin.

Belladonna 6c. One dose every three to four hours, or four to six doses every day.

Fits of dry, barking cough. Worse at night. Croup. (See page 92.)

Drosera 6c. One dose every two to four hours.

To follow an attack.

Pertussin 30c. One dose every day for 3 days (see above).

SCARLET FEVER

Prevention and contact during epidemics or after contacts.

Streptococcin 30c. One dose every week for the duration of the epidemic.

Early Stages (see 'Fevers', page 99)

Bright red face, pallor around mouth. Large pupils. Hot, dry skin. Very sore throat.

Belladonna 6c. One dose every two to four hours for 4–6 doses.

Profuse salivation. Sore throat and mouth, offensive breath. Chills and shivering alternating with the fever.

Mercurius Sol. 6c. One dose every three to 4 hours for 4–6 doses.

MUMPS

The severity of the illness varies from mild to severe and so does the swelling of the glands in front of the ears. Occasionally, glands under the lower jaw become swollen.

Do not give acid or tart drinks as they may cause pain in the glands by provoking a sudden flow of saliva.

Complications are rare.

GLANDULAR FEVER (INFECTIOUS MONONUCLEOSIS)

This virus infection can occur in epidemics or as individual cases and affects school children, teenagers and young adults.

It starts generally as tiredness, aching muscles and headache, tender swollen glands and a fever. A sore throat which continues in spite of antibiotic treatment may arouse suspicion of glandular fever. There may be a measles-like rash in the first ten days, and later jaundice and abdominal pains.

The general picture is very vague and difficult to diagnose, and confirmation may only be possible with special blood tests.

Some patients may be ill for several weeks, with episodes of great debility, sweats and fever occurring for many months.

Treatment

The patient must be kept in bed during the times of fever and must rest at other times, and avoid any strenuous exercise.

(See 'Fevers', page 99)

MUMPS

Prevention and contact.	**Parotidinum 30c.** Three doses in 24 hours.

Early Stage (see 'Fevers', page 99)

Established Stage

Severe headache.	**Pilocarpine Mur. 3x.** One dose every two to four hours for 4–6 doses.
Afterwards.	**Pulsatilla 30c.** One dose twice a day for 3–4 days.

Pilocarpine Mur. 3x will need to be ordered specially from a homoeopathic chemist.

GLANDULAR FEVER (INFECTIOUS MONONUCLEOSIS)

Early Stages (see 'Fevers', page 99)

Prevention – when the child has been in contact with a confirmed case or during an outbreak at the school or in the district.	**Glandular Fever Nosode 30c.** One dose every day for 3 days, and then once a week for a month.
Weakness and debility. Headache, drowsiness. Muscular pains. Ulcerated throat, painful, difficulty swallowing. Enlarged glands. Blotchy rash.	**Ailanthus Gland. 6c.** One dose three times a day until improvement is maintained.

SLEEPLESSNESS

This is frequently caused by overexcitement in the evening, playing too late, television, and a general lack of calm preparation for bed. Noise in the home and the neighbourhood contributes to disturbance.

Obviously, in a persisting case, all these aspects must be attended to. The child should be put to bed as tranquilly as possible. A warm drink, story-telling, a darkened room in the summer and a small night light in the winter, a warm, cosy bed with a favourite soft toy or doll, and not too much attention to the actual problem, may all help to induce sleep.

There are no homoeopathic remedies which act as sedatives, but there are several remedies which may help in particular circumstances.

SLEEPLESSNESS

Anxiety, restlessness. Fear and excitement.	**Aconite 30c.** One to two doses in the evening and on retiring.
Nightmares. Red face, hot dry skin. Pupils dilated, eyes bright. Head hot.	**Belladonna 6c.** One to two doses in the evening and on retiring.
Can't stop thinking. Excitement, happy events. Very sensitive to noise.	**Coffea Cruda 6c.** One to two doses in the evening and on retiring.
Anxiety about forthcoming events (e.g. examinations) or starting a new school.	**Argentum Nit. 6c.** One dose in the evening and on retiring.
Nightmares in a very sensitive child. Fear of dark.	**Phosphorus 6c.** One to two doses in the evening and on retiring.
Very restless – gets out of bed and walks about; tries to sleep in a chair or another bed. Increasingly apprehensive.	**Arsenicum Alb. 6c.** One to two doses in the evening and on retiring.
Restless, miserable, depressed, afraid to be alone. Weepy and hysterical.	**Ignatia 6c.** One to two doses in the evening and on retiring.
Sensitive, mentally active, irritable and angry.	**Nux Vomica 6c.** One to two doses in the evening and on retiring.
Over-sensitive, especially to pain; peevish and petulant.	**Chamomilla 6c.** One to two doses in the evening and on retiring.

SORE THROAT
(Infected Tonsils, Tonsillitis, Pharyngitis)

Sudden Onset (The common sore throat of childhood)

When it comes on suddenly, it is frequently the only complaint apart from a possible raised temperature. Do not forget the basic treatments of:
- Rest – in bed if necessary.
- Fluids – plenty of them.
- Soft, easily swallowed foods.
- In the case of young children particularly, tepid sponging to bring the temperature down to comfortable levels. For older children, a good method is to allow them to play with toys in the bath while it cools down slowly.

Slow Onset

The early symptoms will be of a much more general type and will be the main indications for choosing your homoeopathic remedy.

SORE THROAT
(Infected Tonsils, Tonsillitis, Pharyngitis)

Sudden Onset (The common sore throat of childhood)

Fever, Throat burning, smarting, dry, tingling, bright red. Hurts to swallow.

Aconite 30c. One dose every two to three hours for 3–4 doses.

Throat *red* and glossy, swallowing painful and may spread to the ears. Very hot, dry skin, red face.

Belladonna 6c. One dose every two to three hours and reduce with improvement.

Throat red-raw, sore and smarting. Tongue swollen and coated yellow, indented by teeth. Great salivation but thirsty. Breath smells.

Mercurius Sol. 6c. One dose every two to three hours and reduce with improvement.

Dark red, sore, full feeling. Each swallow causes pain to ears. Difficulty swallowing even water. Neck muscles stiff.

Phytolacca 6c. One dose every two to three hours and reduce with improvement.

Slow Onset

Comes on slowly in humid weather. Heavy head. Neck and shoulders sore. Aching back with shivers up and down. Not very thirsty.

Gelsemium 6c. One dose three to four times a day for 2–4 days.

Previous 'cold'. 'Fishbone' or 'crumb' sensation. Throat very sensitive to touch. Irritable and sensitive to draughts.

Hepar Sulph. 6c. One dose three to four times a day for 2–4 days.

Frequent sore throats. Slowly developing sore throat. Tonsils and glands in neck always enlarged.

Baryta Carb. 6c. One dose three to four times a day for 5–10 days.

TRAVEL SICKNESS

This is a distressing condition which affects many children and some adults. It may vary from simple nausea and headaches to profuse vomiting and collapse.

Anxiety and excitement may play a part in the cause of travel sickness, especially in children, and being confined to the stuffy cabin of the vehicle may also be an important factor. Other people find that the fumes of fuel and exhausts and the smell of cooking or tobacco smoke make matters worse. Most of all, it is the actual motion of the transport and the sensitivity of the patient to the particular type of motion which is the main cause.

Prevention

Anxiety and excitement can be treated before the journey as soon as the symptoms show themselves, even if this is two or three days before. (See 'Anxiety', page 116.)

One or two doses of the remedy either for anxiety or for travel sickness may be given in the hour before the journey starts.

Treatment

Maintain a flow of fresh air during the journey. Provide children with games to take their minds off unpleasant symptoms. Allow for frequent stops during car journeys.

TRAVEL SICKNESS

Anxiety Before the Journey
(See also 'Anxiety', page 117)

**Gelsemium 6c, Ignatia 6c,
Argentum Nitricum 6c**

Over-excitement
Effects of Excitement

Coffea Cruda 6c

The remedy for anxiety or over-excitement may be alternated with the remedy for travel sickness, if necessary.

The Journey

Nausea, vomiting, saliva increased. Metallic taste in mouth. Worse thinking of food. Much worse on sight or smell of food. Giddiness, and must lie down. Improved by warmth.

Cocculus 6c. One or two doses before the journey and on the return of any symptoms during the journey.

Nausea, vomiting and giddiness. Very pale, cold sweats, fainting. Collapse. Worse with smell of tobacco smoke. Headache like a band around the head. Improved by cold.

Tabacum 6c. One or two doses before, and one repeated during the journey.

Nausea with greatly increased saliva. Empty feeling relieved by food. Vomiting and giddiness worse with noise. Headache in the neck and back of head. Improved by closing eyes.

Petroleum 6c. One or two doses before, and one repeated during the journey.

Throughout the book I normally indicate the use of a single remedy. But this can be difficult to find, especially in confusing social situations such as modern travel. If you are in doubt about the remedy, alternate the two most likely ones as the symptoms begin to return.

— NOTES —

GENERAL PROBLEMS

ACNE VULGARIS
(Blackheads, Pustules, 'Blind boils')

This is a common skin condition in adolescents, caused by an imbalance in the hormone levels. It can occur later, particularly in women pre-menstrually, or occasionally with hormone changes during or after pregnancy or in the menopause. Some patients find that a fatty or too rich diet worsens the condition.

The spots themselves are caused by inflammation, with or without secondary infection, setting up in small sebaceous glands of the skin which have become blocked up. They may or may not be painful.

External Treatment

This should be as gentle as possible. Harsh scouring or 'strong' antiseptic soaps and ointments should be avoided. Creams and ointments containing antibiotics or the cortisone type of hormones **should not** be used, since general allergic reactions and permanent damage to the skin can easily occur.

ACNE VULGARIS
(Blackheads, Pustules, 'Blind boils')

Blackheads with an oily skin. Small pimples on face and forehead.	**Selenium 6c.** One dose morning and evening.
Painful burning and stinging. *Pustules* on the face, chest, shoulder. 'Blind boils'.	**Kali Brom. 6c.** One dose morning and evening.
Painful red pustules with discharging yellow pus.	**Hepar Sulph. 6c.** One dose morning and evening.

Try the most appropriate remedy listed above for three to six weeks. If only partially effective, or not effective, consult a homoeopath. Since acne is the result in the skin of a general bodily disturbance, other deeper-acting constitutional remedies may be needed.

External Treatment

Infected areas or individual spots may be helped by applying a little **Calendula** cream or ointment. If the skin is greasy, dabbing on a little of the Tincture of Calendula may be better.

ANXIETY
(Anxiety state, Tension state, 'Being up-tight')

(See also 'Fear', page 138)

Sudden short-lived anxiety due to particular circumstances is natural and needs no treatment, since after a short time the mind and body return to normal. However, with repeated episodes of acute fear and anxiety, or long-continued unrelieved anxiety, a state of 'chronic anxiety' develops. A 'chronic anxiety state' is a complex condition and does not fall within the scope of this book.

If you have been taking transquillisers for many months or even years, you must realise that it can be **very dangerous** if such drugs are stopped suddenly. Violent reactions both physical and mental can occur. Evaluation and treatment from a homoeopathic doctor is advisable in such cases.

The homoeopathic remedies described on the opposite page differ a little from most of the others in this book because they try, very briefly, to indicate the wider aspects of the remedies and of the type of patient they are most likely to help. This, when fully developed, is called the 'constitutional approach'. It assesses the relative importance of psychological, physical, dietary, climatic and social aspects of the whole person. Generally speaking, you will not need this approach when dealing in a First Aid way with your family.

When possible stressful situations should be avoided. When this cannot be done, one must learn, by whatever means possible, to be less affected by stress. Most people try to avoid changing any established patterns of living and thinking. Remedies alone should not be expected to compensate for the bad habits of a lifetime.

ANXIETY
(Anxiety state, Tension state, 'Being up-tight')

(See also 'Fear', page 139, and indications for Gelsemium, Argentum Nitricum and Aconite)

Easily anxious and discouraged. Apprehensive with palpitations. Forgetful and confused. Obstinate and slow. Flabby, chilly, dislikes activity.

Calcarea Carb. 30c. One dose two to three times a day for a few days, and reduce with improvement.

Over-sensitive. Easily fearful. Fears the dark. Needs reassurance. Restless and fidgety. Bright, emotional, loving.

Phosphorus 30c. One dose two to three times a day for a few days, and reduce with improvement.

Over-sensitive – sighing. Problems exaggerated. Over-reaction – palpitations. Insomnia, loss of appetite. Easily distracted into an improvement.

Ignatia 30c. One dose two to three times a day, when needed. Can be used before particular events.

Marked lack of confidence. Fears failure – covers up. Irritable and touchy. Hates contradiction.

Lycopodium 30c. One dose two to three times a day, and reduce with improvement.

Very chilly, thin and weak. Nervous, irritable, stubborn. Anxiety before events. Fears failure. Exhausted by effort.

Silica 30c. One dose two to three times a day, and reduce with improvement.

CHILBLAINS AND POOR CIRCULATION

'Poor Circulation' is a loose term that explains a range of conditions from cold hands and feet, 'dead fingers', blotchy mottled legs, painful cramps and chilblains.

Chilblains can occur on the ears, the fingers and the toes. They can be described as the damage done to the tissues from a spasm of the blood vessels triggered off by the cold. An occasional episode can be treated on a first-aid basis, but recurring episodes or a lifelong problem indicate a constitutional weakness. A rather special condition called Reynaud's disease is characterised by blue or white fingers triggered by the cold, especially by placing the hands in cold water. In any of these circumstances consult an experienced homoeopath. If the condition gets worse, consult your own doctor in all cases because special investigations may be needed.

Prevention

- Stimulate the circulation by plenty of exercise.
- Hands, ears and feet should not be needlessly exposed to cold and must be protected appropriately by warm clothing and boots.
- Homoeopathic remedies can be effective in prevention. Use the remedy which may have been helpful in the previous winter. If you are new to homoeopathy use a remedy chosen on the symptoms you remember. Take one dose every week, starting at the beginning of winter, but if symptoms arise, check that you are using the right remedy and then follow the dosage on the opposite page.

CHILBLAINS AND POOR CIRCULATION

Poor Circulation

Cold hands and feet. 'Blue' or 'dead white' fingers and toes. Pain and cramps. Burning helped by cold.

Secale 6c. One dose morning and evening. Continue for several weeks at a time.

Cramps and burning pain helped by heat. Cold hands and feet.

Arsenicum Alb. 6c. One dose morning and evening. Continue for several weeks at a time.

Cramps – especially at night in old people. Coldness of hands and feet. Blotchy blue skin. Cramp of the *calves* and *feet*.

Cuprum Met. 6c. One dose morning and evening, or one dose each night on retiring.

Chilblains

Red swellings. Pustules. Burning, itching and prickling. Worse when cold.

Agaricus 6c. One dose morning and evening until relief.

Blue blotches. Stabbing pain. Worse with heat. Better for cold and exercise.

Pulsatilla 6c. One dose morning and evening until relief.

COLITIS

This term covers a range of problems with recurring diarrhoea, spasms of pain, perhaps blood and mucus, and occasionally mild fever and malaise. Sometimes normal motions or small constipated ones may be passed.

Recurring symptoms like these must first be investigated by a specialist at a hospital. It is necessary to exclude more serious disease. There might be, on the one hand, infection by germs or parasites (usually contracted during travels outside Europe), which can be quickly and safely treated by orthodox medication; on the other hand, there might be a condition better treated by surgery.

There are four conditions which come under the heading of colitis and which have some symptoms in common. These are called irritable colon, spastic colon, mucous colitis and ulcerative colitis.

Irritable colon is a condition where there is overactivity of an otherwise normal bowel. There are bouts of diarrhoea or an increased frequency of normal bowel motions, with or without pain. These bouts are usually related to stressful emotions, overtiredness and mental and physical overactivity.

Spastic colon is characterised by very painful spasms of the colon, which are brought on by foods or laxatives. The spasms may be relieved by passing wind or passing a stool.

Mucous colitis is a condition where motions are covered in clear mucus, or joined together by mucous strands, or where large lumps of mucus are passed alone.

If any of the above three diagnoses have been made after investigation by the hospital specialist, and orthodox treatment has been only partially successful, then the homoeopathic remedies on the page opposite may be helpful on a first-aid basis. If the remedies are themselves only partially successful, the advice of a homoeopath must be sought.

Ulcerative colitis is a potentially dangerous condition, where there may be pain, fever, profuse diarrhoea with varying amounts of blood and mucus, marked loss of weight and general debility and ill health. **First-aid treatment has no part to play here. The patient must be in the care of a physician**. If the patient wishes to have homoeopathic treatment at the same time it must be guided by a very experienced homoeopath.

COLITIS

Anxiety or fears, expecially in anticipation of an event. Loose motions.	**Argentum Nit. 6c.** One dose every one to two hours during a bout, or
	Gelsemium 6c. One dose one to three hours before an event.
Loose motions every morning, and more likely to be with spasms of pain.	**Ignatia 6c.** One dose each morning, or one each morning and evening.
Painless repeated diarrhoea. Distension and tenderness of abdomen. Rumbling. General weakness.	**China 6c.** One dose three to four times a day, best before meals.
Sudden cramp-like pains improved by bending double or by applying a hot water bottle to the abdomen. Worse after food and drinks.	**Colocynthis 6c.** One dose every 15–30 minutes until eased.
Spasms of pain after emotional crises. May have diarrhoea.	**Ignatia 6c.** One dose every 15–30 minutes until eased.
Stools liquid but containing hard lumps. Tongue coated white. Belching undigested food.	**Antimonium Crud. 6c.** One dose three times a day, reducing with improvement.
Dry, bulky motions covered in mucus or joined together by strings of mucus. Windy pains. Offensive gas.	**Graphites 6c.** One dose three times a day, reducing with improvement.

COMMON COLD – EARLY STAGES

Colds and influenza are infectious illnesses caused by viruses. There are many types and they vary from year to year.

The resistance of the individual to these viruses is of great importance and this depends on good general health. General health, in its turn, depends upon high-quality nourishing foods, adequate rest and recreation, the absence of prolonged or severe stress and daily physical exercise. A deficiency of any of these can weaken the health as a whole, and the person becomes prone to illness.

Homoeopathic treatment can be used to improve the resistance to infection. Well-selected remedies will speed up the cure and reduce the development of catarrh, sinusitis and bronchitis.

See also the discussions in the section on Children's Problems: 'Colds and Influenza' – pages 84–7, 'Fever' – page 99, 'Cough' – page 90, 'Sore Throat' – page 108.

General Management

- Go home and stay away from other people, if possible. This is important during the first day or so when you are very infectious.
- Take extra vitamin C – up to 500mg twice a day – especially if you have a temperature.
- Choose a remedy from the list opposite and change it if the symptoms change. If you cannot decide which is the better of two remedies take them alternately at intervals of one hour.

COMMON COLD – EARLY STAGES

Prevention

'Cold and Flu tablets'. One tablet morning and evening on the first (and perhaps also the 15th) day of each month.

Early Stages

Very first signs of a cold. Sudden chill, shivering. Fever.

Aconite 30c. One dose every two hours, for the first day – into the second day or overnight.

Very sore raw nostrils and upper lip caused by profusely running nose. Sneezing. Painless watery eyes.

Allium Cepa 6c. One dose every two hours until improvement, and then reduce.

Eyes red and sore from burning tears. Profuse watery nasal discharge. Sneezing.

Euphrasia 6c. One dose every two hours until improvement, and then reduce.

Sudden intense chill with shivering. Unable to get warm. Patient irritable. Nose dry and stuffed up.

Nux Vomica 6c. One dose every two hours until improvement, and then reduce.

Stiff neck and pain in the throat, back and limbs. Eyes and nose streaming. Sneezing. Brought on by being chilled when hot, or drenched in cold wet weather.

Dulcamara 6c. One dose every two hours until improvement, and then reduce.

If the chosen remedy does not relieve your symptoms within twenty-four hours it is probable that it is not the correct one. Reassess the symptoms at this stage and make a further choice.

COMMON COLD – LATER STAGES

As a rule people tend to follow their own patterns in the way that a cold develops. Occasionally a particular type of infection will impose its own pattern on the patient.

From the homoeopathic point of view this does not matter – you choose the remedy by matching the main symptoms of the patient and the remedy.

The tendency is for the watery discharge of the early cold to become secondarily infected. Yellow or green catarrh develops at this point, and can be thick and difficult to dislodge. The infection may spread to the chest or to the throat or ears.

General Management

- Avoid over-exposure to bad weather and avoid other people with infections.
- Take it easy for a few days – give the body a chance to throw off the whole illness.
- Use steam inhalations to help the catarrh to disperse, but do not use strong-smelling substances like Oil of Eucalyptus or Wintergreen or Friar's Balsam. These may antidote the effects of the homoeopathic remedies you are taking.
- Continue to change the remedies as the symptoms change.

COMMON COLD – LATER STAGES

'Flu-like cold'. Heavy head, tired heavy eyes. Backache with shivers up and down. Arms and legs ache. Sore nose. Wants to lie down and sleep.

Gelsemium 6c. One dose at intervals of one to two hours and reduce with improvement.

Pain over the eyes. Stinging, watery nasal discharge. Violent sneezing. Smarting, watering eyes.

Kali Iod. 6c. One dose at intervals of one to two hours and reduce with improvement.

Thick, yellow, burning nasal discharge. Nostrils may be raw and ulcerated. Profuse sweating or chilled and shivering even in a hot room. Offensive breath.

Merc. Sol. 6c. One dose at intervals of one to two hours and reduce with improvement.

Thick, sticky, yellow or green nasal discharge. May be bloodstained, difficult to blow out. Thick, sticky crusts in nose.

Kali Bich. 6c. One dose at intervals of one to two hours and reduce with improvement.

Stringy, yellow nasal discharge, sticky and difficult to shift. Post-nasal drip.

Hydrastis 6c. One dose at intervals of one to two hours and reduce with improvement.

CONSTIPATION

It is now recognised that it is healthy to have two or three soft motions daily. A person is constipated when he or she repeatedly fails to have a regular bowel action. The motion may be large and bulky, either soft or hard, but it may also be small lumps more or less crammed together. The basic fact is that the bowel is not cleared on a regular basis.

Many people become constipated because they never develop the habit of going to the toilet as soon as they feel the urge to move their bowels. In this way 'the urge' gradually becomes weaker – and the bowels are moved less frequently and eventually the retention of bowel contents results.

It is a mistake to resort to laxatives, and prevention is better than cure.

You must consult your doctor if the constipation has been getting worse over several weeks or months, or if you have used laxatives regularly and now find that you need more to achieve the same result.

You should also consult your doctor if the constipated motion is passed with blood or mucus, or if piles develop and increase in severity.

General Management

- Increase the amount of 'roughage' in the diet. This is best done by eating wholemeal bread and cereals and by increasing the quantity of fruit and vegetables eaten daily. At the same time, eliminate highly-refined and manufactured foods; in short, cut out 'junk food' and eat a 'whole food' diet.
- Drink more liquids throughout the day. You should aim at about three pints of liquid of one sort or another in twenty-four hours. Obviously, you should drink more if you perspire profusely because of hot weather or hard exercise.
- Establish a regular time to go to the toilet.
- Use the appropriate remedy on the opposite page. If there is doubt about the most suitable remedy, take Nux Vomica 6c each evening and Sulphur 6c each morning for several days.

CONSTIPATION

Soft, sticky, unformed stool. No urge to use the bowels. Loss of expulsive power. Straining with great effort.

Alumina 6c. One dose morning and evening until improvement.

Stools small, hard, dry balls which may be packed together. No urge to use the bowels. Poor appetite.

Opium 6c. One dose morning and evening until improvement.

Small, variable stools. Frequent, ineffective urging with feeling of incomplete emptying. Lack of regular bowel habits. Over-use of laxatives in the past.

Nux Vomica 6c. One dose morning and evening until improvement.

Stools large, hard and difficult to expel – they seem to slip back. Spasm of muscles of the anus. Worse during menstrual periods.

Silica 6c. One dose morning and evening until improvement.

Small, hard, dry stools. Great effort with pain and burning. Constipation may alternate with diarrhoea.

Sulphur 6c. One dose morning and evening until improvement.

COUGH

Coughing is due to irritation in the respiratory tract at any point between the larynx (voice box) and the deeper parts of the lungs.

A cough may flare up suddenly, caused by dust, fumes or smoke. Usually it occurs as part of an overall picture of a throat or chest infection. The chest infection may have developed from 'a cold' or it may have started 'on the chest'.

However, for the purposes of a book such as this, coughs can be divided into three main groups, (although there is likely to be an overlapping of symptoms). These are:

- Dry, hacking cough – e.g. laryngitis.
- Spasmodic, repetitive coughs – e.g. whooping coughs.
- Loose coughs, with phlegm or sputum – e.g. bronchitis.

General Management

The patient should avoid places where the cough is worsened, such as dusty or smoky places, or very cold, damp weather outside. If the general condition is not improving, he or she should stay indoors, or even go to bed, or use inhalations of steam. The latter must be carefully supervised, to prevent scalding.

Call the doctor if:

- The overall condition worsens.
- There are other problems, such as diabetes or a heart condition.
- The new infection is in addition to a long-term chest infection such as chronic bronchitis or emphysema.

Do not attempt to treat severe bronchitis or pneumonia yourself. The doctor may have to prescribe an antibiotic, which at some stage could be in the best interest of the patient.

If you cannot decide which of two remedies is the more appropriate in the circumstances, take them alternately, as often as is necessary for relief. Remember to change the remedy with a change in the symptom picture.

COUGH

Dry Cough

Croup-like cough in very dry, cold weather. Anxiety and restlessness. Fever, thirst, no sweating.

Aconite 30c. One dose at fifteen minute intervals, reducing with improvement.

Rough, noisy croup-like cough. Sudden onset in cold weather. Better in a warm, steamy room.

Hepar Sulph. 6c. One dose at fifteen minute intervals, reducing with improvement.

Raw, tearing, burning pain in a croup-like cough. Improves with hot drinks.

Spongia 6c. One dose at fifteen minute intervals, reducing with improvement.

Slow, gradual fever; irritation of air passages. Cough worse for movement and entering a warm room; can be worse at night. Much thirst for cold drinks. Stabbing pains in throat or chest.

Bryonia 6c. One dose at fifteen minute intervals, reducing with improvement.

Spasmodic Cough

Bouts of dry cough – a bit like whooping cough. Worse at night and lying down. May be wheezing; occasionally croup-like.

Drosera 6c. One dose at fifteen minute intervals, reducing with improvement.

Crowing spasmodic cough. Better sipping cold water.

Cuprum Met. 6c. One dose at fifteen minute intervals, reducing with improvement.

Spasms of coughing; the more he coughs, the more he has to.

Ignatia 6c. One dose morning and evening and after a bout of coughing.

Loose Cough

Spasmodic cough, worse in open air. Breathless. Rapid development of phlegm which may be vomited up.

Ipecacuanha 6c. One dose four to six times a day, reducing with improvement.

Thick yellow loose phlegm. Runny nose. Cough productive in day and dry at night. Better in fresh air. Towards end of illness.

Pulsatilla 6c. One dose four to six times a day, reducing with improvement.

Loose phlegm, thick and difficult to cough up. Breathless. Wheezing, noisy chest.

Antimonium Tart. 6c. One dose four to six times a day, reducing with improvement.

CYSTITIS

This is a painful condition of the bladder which causes painful urination, with frequency during the day and often disturbed nights. There may also be incontinence, urgency and very painful bladder spasms.

Cystitis is usually caused by infection and can be treated homoeopathically very successfully although in some cases antibiotic treatment may be necessary. If this happens, homoeopathic remedies can be used as well, and the need for prolonged antibiotic treatment may be reduced or eliminated.

Caution

There are other causes for these symptoms. The patient with more than one episode of acute cystitis **must** consult the family doctor, with a view to full investigation of the urinary tract as a whole. Provided that serious disease has been excluded by the appropriate medical tests, homoeopathic medicine may be more beneficial than some orthodox medical treatments.

CYSTITIS

Stinging, burning pain before, during and after urinating. Very frequent. Small quantities of dark urine with or without blood.

Cantharis 6c. One dose at intervals of thirty minutes to one hour – reduce with improvement.

Frequency, urgency. Very painful spasms of bladder. Burning pain with little or no urine. Dark bloody urine.

Mercurius Corr. 6c. One dose at intervals of thirty minutes to one hour – reduce with improvement.

Frequency, unbearable pain at end. Urination easier standing. Urine scanty, deposits blood.

Sarsaparilla 6c. One dose at intervals of thirty minutes to one hour – reduce with improvement.

Frequency with much urine. Pain *during* and *after* completion. Bladder feels weary between urination. Bed wetting in children.

Equisetum 6c. One dose three to four times a day – reduce with improvement.

'Honeymoon' cystitis in women. Burning pains in the urethra, especially between urinating. Pain better passing urine.

Staphysagria 6c. One dose twice a day for one week.

Staphysagria can be used on a regular basis for those women who suffer urethritis/cystitis each time after intercourse. Take three times a week, or following intercourse.

Frequency, leaking. Dribbling. Difficulty in starting. Incontinence.

Causticum 30c. One dose two to three times a day.

DENTAL ABSCESS (GUM BOILS)

In this condition an abscess has formed at some point around a tooth; that is, pus is forming a 'gum boil'. A dentist must be consulted and will probably prescribe an antibiotic before operating to drain the abscess.

Before this, the most suitable homoeopathic remedy on the opposite page will greatly help the condition. It can be used together with an antibiotic, if prescribed.

After the dental procedure, the dentist may advise 'hot salt mouth washes' as frequently as possible. This is a good initial cleansing procedure, but it is only necessary to do this two or three times. Afterwards, use a mouth wash made up of 5–10 drops of Calendula or Hypercal tincture in a glass of cool, previously boiled water.

DENTAL ABSCESS (GUM BOILS)

Any of the remedies listed on page 167 for toothache may be helpful. The following remedies may also be of value.

Oral Treatment

Rubbed over the swelling as frequently as needed.

Hypericum tincture, Hypercal tincture: every two to three hours.

By Mouth

Throbbing, hot, shining, swelling. May have malaise and headache. Usually before pus is obvious.

Belladonna 6c. One dose every hour.

Early swelling, but pus not ready to discharge. To speed up abscess formation.

Hepar Sulph. 6c. One dose every hour.

Pus discharging. Unwell. Foul taste.

Pyrogen 6c. One dose every two to four hours for 3–5 days.

DIARRHOEA

Sudden Onset

This term refers to the passing of very loose or watery motions which may contain blood, slime or, on occasion, pieces of undigested food, and which may smell offensive. Usually it is caused by infection from food or water, or by overeating fruit or unusual foods. All of these can occur on holiday in hot sunny countries.

The homoeopathic remedies on the opposite page should prove helpful for these situations. For the traveller and holiday maker, Arsenicum Album (or failing that, Veratrum Album) will probably be the most usual remedies. If the diarrhoea persists, then one of the other remedies listed might be more appropriate, and the use of a 'Kaolin mixture' can also be helpful. Antibiotics are not helpful in general, and too often bring about a reactive diarrhoea and other complications.

In very hot weather, old people and children can dehydrate rapidly. This must be prevented by giving frequent drinks.

In nervous adults and in children, diarrhoea can arise from fears and anxiety. Here the answer is to treat the person as a whole in relation to the type of anxiety. (See also 'Fear' – page 138 and 'Anxiety' – page 116.)

Caution

If the acute bouts and pains of diarrhoea recur at intervals of weeks or months, or if there is blood or slime in the motions, or if the patient loses weight and is generally unwell, it is **essential** that you consult your doctor for further investigation.

DIARRHOEA

Sudden Onset

Severe watery, burning and stinging diarrhoea. Chill, weakness, anxiety or prostration. Usually vomiting, but thirsty for small drinks. Can be worse after midnight. Food poisoning. Travellers' diarrhoea. Contaminated water.

Arsenicum Alb. 6c. One dose every two to three hours and reduce with improvement, or one dose after each motion.

Great nausea not helped by vomiting. Motion smelly, frothy yellow or green. Colicky pain and straining. Diarrhoea in spasms. No thirst, clean tongue.

Ipecacuanha 6c. One dose every two to three hours and reduce with improvement, or one dose after each motion.

Great weakness and vomiting. Bitter taste, hungry with no appetite. Painful, windy rumbling; distension. Diarrhoea with wind, worse after fruit and milk.

China 6c. One dose every two to three hours and reduce with improvement, or one dose after each bout of diarrhoea.

Severe, gushing watery diarrhoea; rumbling of wind; ill-smelling. Worse in morning. Colicky pains before; urging after. Weak feeling after. Pain improved by heat and by lying on abdomen.

Podophyllum 6c. One dose every two to three hours and reduce with improvement, or one dose after each motion.

Painful cramps, which start and finish suddenly. Improvement by bending double, by heat and by strong pressure.

Colocynthis 6c. One dose every two to three hours and reduce with improvement, or one dose after each motion.

ECZEMA

This is the name given to many different conditions of the skin, from dry flaking to moist, oozing and sometimes cracking and bleeding skin. The affected area of skin frequently itches severely. This can cause distressing loss of sleep, with irritability and loss of efficiency at work or school. Scratching can introduce infections with further complications, and if continued over a long time can cause an unhealthy thickening of the skin.

The cause of eczema is a breakdown in the defence mechanisms of the body resulting in an allergic or sensitivity reaction. There can be great variation in how long the condition lasts. Stress may cause it to flare up.

Babies developing 'infantile eczema' may have been allergic to cows' milk protein in bottle feeds or to 'foreign' protein in immunisation injections. Usually there will be relations within the family who have allergic conditions like asthma, hay fever, 'dermatitis', or very specific allergies to certain foods or chemicals in make-up or detergents.

The remedies given on the page opposite are intended for first-aid only. It is essential that long-term treatment should only be undertaken by an experienced homoeopath.

External Treatment

Avoid using applications containing antibiotics and cortisone-type of drugs as much as possible. However, in severe situations, remember that medical advice must be taken and corticosteroid preparations may in fact be life-saving.

Dry eczema may be helped better by applying soothing, bland cream or ointment, for example, **Urtica Urens** cream, depending upon the patient's individual response.

Weeping and infected eczemas are probably best treated by **Calendula** lotion. Using freshly prepared lotion (5–10 drops in half a pint of previously boiled water), moisten (and keep moist) applications of sterile gauze squares. These should be changed less frequently as the condition improves. Occasionally **Graphites** ointment can be helpful.

Itching may be helped by **Paeonia** ointment or **Urtica** ointment.

ECZEMA

Dry Eczema

Hot, sweaty patient with rough itching skin. Some patches of infection. Irritation worse with washing and heat of the bed.

Sulphur 6c. One dose on alternate days for a week and then one every day. N.B. *Stop if there is a reaction, wait for it to settle and then recommence treatment.*

Dry red itching areas, especially on hands, wrists and in the bends of joints. Generally eased by warmth and much worse in cold, damp weather. Small blisters.

Rhus Tox. 6c. One dose a day for a week and then one dose morning and evening until improvement is maintained.

Unwashed, grey, greasy skin. Eczema at bends of knees and elbows. Irritation worse with cold. Patient chilly also.

Psorinum 6c. One dose morning and evening. Stop with improvement.

Moist Eczema

Oozing, clear or yellow discharge; 'honey-like'. Any area, but common behind ears and on the head.

Graphites 6c. One dose morning and evening.

Continue the treatment until an improvement is established, and then stop. If the eczema seems to be starting again, start the treatment again.

FEAR

Fear is a serious symptom and is usually an obvious response to an obvious cause. In certain cases no cause is obvious. Sometimes the fear is not simply a sudden reaction, but a recurring one when presented with the same situation. It is then known as a 'phobic anxiety state', e.g. claustrophobia or agoraphobia. In other cases the fear seems like a continuous state of heightened anxiety.

The homoeopathic remedies on the page opposite will, if chosen correctly, help in the management of the condition; other measures, such as psychotherapy, may also be required. Certainly, a long-established problem will have to be very carefully assessed by a homoeopath before starting treatment. Treatment may take months to be effective.

With minor difficulties, such as stage fright or examination nerves, the remedy can be given on going to bed for a few nights before the event, and on the morning or afternoon of the event itself.

You will notice that the potencies suggested are higher than usual. Use the 30c potency first, and if this is not entirely successful ask your chemist to get the 200c potency for you. In case of difficulty, any of the organisations listed on pages 178–9 can give you the addresses of homoeopathic chemists who supply by post.

FEAR

Sudden panic, terror or shock. Can be 'out of the blue'. Agitated, nightmares. Can over-breathe and produce palpitations and numbness, or tingling sensations in the cheeks, hands or feet.

Aconite 30c or **200c.** One dose immediately and repeat at fifteen minute intervals up to 3 or 4 times if necessary.

Give after acute shocks or accidents

Arnica 30c

Apprehension before an event; 'Exam nerves' or 'Stage fright'. Panic in a crowd, lift, tube station. Agitated. Patient moves rapidly.

Argentum Nit. 30c or **200c.** One dose before the event if possible or repeat as necessary.

Dread – unaccountable fear. Physical and mental restlessness. Fears being alone, especially late at night.

Arsenicum Alb. 30c or **200c.** One dose immediately and repeat every half hour if necessary.

Trembling weakness, 'paralysed by fear'. 'All of a dither'. Mind blank, can't speak or think. 'Exam nerves', 'Stage fright'.

Gelsemium 30c or **200c.** One dose before the event if possible or repeat as necessary.

Persisting fear. Fear returning after remembering the fear-inducing event.

Opium 30c or **200c.** One dose at the time and repeat every day for 3–4 days.

HAY FEVER

This seems to be an increasingly common condition during the summer. It is due to a sensitivity or allergy to the pollens of trees, shrubs, flowers and grasses and, occasionally, to the spores of fungi. Generally the problem is related to part of the season, but sometimes it may spread from spring through the summer and on to the autumn.

The symptoms may vary from year to year, may or may not be affected by the weather or the pollen count, and may get steadily worse, or fade away.

The usual picture of hay fever is one of sneezing with either a blocked or runny nose, red itching and watering eyes, or itching at the back of the nose or throat or in the ears. There may occasionally be a tightness of the chest or even asthma, and more rarely still, an actual fever.

The treatment of the underlying cause of the sensitivity may be very complex and needs the help of a homoeopath if the cure is to be permanent.

The remedies on the page opposite are a few of the most helpful ones which can be used as first aid. If you are not able to choose a remedy accurately, or if your choice is not effective, alternate the two remedies which seem to be nearest to the symptoms of the patient.

HAY FEVER

Bouts of sneezing. Burning, watery nasal discharge. Sore nostrils and upper lip. Eyes itching, painless watering. Tickling cough.

Allium Cepa 6c. One dose 2–4 times a day.

Bouts of sneezing. Profuse, watery nasal discharge. Numbness and itching of the throat. (Patient tries to scratch it with the back of the tongue). Very sensitive to strong scents. Sinus pains over the eyes. Sensation of lump in throat – needs to swallow.

Sabadilla 6c. One dose 2–4 times a day.

Itching eyes. Itching roof of mouth and back of throat. Itching deep in the ears. Itching nostrils. Sneezing – loss of smell.

Arundo 6c. One dose 2–4 times a day.

Sneezing (violent). Cough. Nose running, or burning and dry. Eyes hot. Heavy, swollen eyelids. Throat tingling, dry and burning. Face flushed and heavy-looking.

Gelsemium 6c. One dose 2–4 times a day.

Sneezing, watery nose (but not sore). Eyes red, burning tears, swollen lids. Dislikes bright light. General headache.

Euphrasia 6c. One dose 2–4 times a day.

Loss of sense of smell. Nose itching, stuffy and obstructed and unable to clear by blowing. Nostrils and upper lip sore.

Ammonium Mur. 6c. One dose 2–4 times a day.

One method of treating hay fever is to take one tablet of **Mixed Pollens 30c** each day. Many patients find that this remedy clears up the symptoms completely, while most find them much reduced. However, there are some patients whose improvement only begins when they stop taking the remedy, having taken it for a week or two. The improvement may last for several weeks.

The remedy **Grass 30c** may be a help to those people who are affected by mowing the lawn. One tablet may be taken before and after mowing.

HEADACHE

Headaches which become more frequent or intense, or which become constant, need medical evaluation. You must consult your doctor, who may refer you to hospital for specialist investigation.

Migraine

A migraine is a headache, usually one-sided, which occurs at certain times of the week or month, or in groups at longer intervals. It may be accompanied by nausea and vomiting.

After investigation by your doctor, such headaches are best treated by a homoeopath, because constitutional treatment will be needed and the assessment is likely to be complex.

The remedies on the opposite page will cover a large proportion of the headaches arising out of everyday situations.

HEADACHE

Congestion with throbbing, brought on by hairdryers or over-exposure to strong sunshine. Worse in stuffy heat, strong light and noise. Flushed red face.

Belladonna 6c. One dose every fifteen to thirty minutes. Reduce with improvement.

Heavy aching in back of head, neck and shoulders. Heavy eyes and drowsy. Better if head held high. Ends with passing large quantities of urine. Drowsy.

Gelsemium 6c. One dose every fifteen to thirty minutes. Reduce with improvement.

Bursting or crushing headache, made worse by any movement of the head or even the eyes. Worse by coughing or straining. Head held still, better with pressure on the head and lying still. Peevish.

Bryonia 6c. One dose every fifteen to thirty minutes. Reduce with improvement.

Nausea and splitting headache. Scalp sore. Can wake with it or after eating. Worse with mental effort. Better with warmth and lying down. Bad-tempered and irritable. Hangover.

Nux Vomica 6c. One dose every fifteen to thirty minutes. Reduce with improvement.

HOARSENESS AND LOSS OF VOICE

Hoarseness and loss of voice are commonly associated with colds and flus and with 'colds going down onto the chest'. Some people suffer more than others, and the problem may occur for no very obvious reason at all. In some occupations involving singing or speaking, hoarseness and loss of voice are an occupational hazard.

The homoeopathic remedies on the page opposite are very much first aid remedies which will help. If the hoarseness persists for more than two to three weeks you should consult your own doctor. He will probably refer you to an Ear, Nose and Throat specialist for investigation to exclude other more serious disease. If nothing serious is found by the specialist, treatment by an experienced homoeopath is likely to be most beneficial.

HOARSENESS AND LOSS OF VOICE

Speaking and singing. Hoarseness at beginning; improves while using voice; hoarseness at end when tired.

Rhus Tox. 6c. One dose fifteen minutes before using voice.

Hoarseness after severe over-use, i.e. shouting, screaming, singing.

Arnica 6c. One dose 2–4 times a day.

Hoarseness with a sensation of rawness in the larynx. Worse with cough, swallowing or speaking. May be thick sputum.

Argentum Met. 6c or **Argentum Nit. 6c.** One dose 2–4 times a day. Reduce with improvement.

Loss of voice after excessive use. Worse in the morning. Raw larynx. Better with cold drinks.

Causticum 6c. One dose 2–4 times a day. Reduce with improvement.

Hoarseness worse in evening and early night. Larynx painful, preventing speech. Dry, tickling cough made worse moving into cold air.

Phosphorus 6c. One dose 2–4 times a day. Reduce with improvement.

Hoarseness, variable. Voice changes pitch. Difficult to control. Hawking phlegm. Better resting. Worse singing and talking.

Arum Triph. 6c. One dose six times a day. Reduce with improvement.

INDIGESTION (DYSPEPSIA)

This is a state of discomfort in the lower chest and upper stomach, with some of the following complaints: a heavy sensation in the stomach after food; actual swelling of the stomach area; bloating – a sensation of swelling with or without flatulence; 'wind' belched up or rumbling around, or trapped and uncomfortable; burping up watery or solid stomach contents; 'acidity – sharp or burning pains in the upper abdomen.

There are many possible combinations of the above symptoms, but acute attacks are short-lived and the cause can usually be avoided (e.g. by not eating particular foods or by eating in a more regular and relaxed way).

Chronic indigestion which has gone on for weeks, months or years should be investigated by your doctor, since treatment is less likely to be by means of simple measures, and there may be a more serious condition underlying the symptom picture.

One of the most common causes of long-lasting or recurring bouts of indigestion is psychological stress – and this is why homoeopathic remedies can be so helpful. On the one hand the psychological factors can be treated in their own right, and on the other hand the same factors can form part of the whole constitutional picture and increase the accuracy of the remedy.

Generally speaking, you will not need this approach when using homoeopathy in a first aid way.

It goes without saying that diet, rest and relaxation must be improved. Where possible, stressful situations should be avoided. When this cannot be done, one must learn, by whatever means possible, to be less affected by stress. Most people try to avoid changing any established patterns of living and thinking. Remedies alone should not be expected to compensate for the bad habits of a lifetime. The remedies on the opposite page may be used at the onset of a bout of indigestion. Vary the frequency of the dose according to the patient's response, increasing the intervals between doses as the patient improves.

The remedies may also be used at a rate of two or three times a day for a few days to treat a more long-standing situation.

INDIGESTION (DYSPEPSIA)

Over-eating. Irritability. Bloated heavy feeling in stomach. Flatulence and heartburn. Sometimes nausea and vomiting. Too much alcohol.

Nux Vomica 6c. One dose at intervals of fifteen to thirty minutes for 2–3 doses.

Great flatulence and bowel rumbling. Unwell if meals missed or delayed. Likes sweet things.

Lycopodium 6c. One dose at intervals of fifteen to thirty minutes for 2–3 doses.

Belching wind and sour taste. Pain in pit of stomach. Generally worse after eating.

Carbo Veg. 6c. One dose at intervals of fifteen to thirty minutes for 2–3 doses.

Heavy weight in stomach immediately after food. Bitter taste. Nausea and pains through to back and shoulders. Headache.

Bryonia 6c. One dose at intervals of fifteen to thirty minutes for 2–3 doses.

Long history of dyspepsia. Sour belching. Constipation and bowel rumbling. Over-eating and over-drinking.

Sulphur 6c. One dose at intervals of fifteen to thirty minutes for 2–3 doses.

Changeable symptoms. Thirstless, coated tongue. Nauseated by fats and rich foods – likes but disagrees. Full, bloated feeling two hours after food.

Pulsatilla 6c. One dose at intervals of fifteen to thirty minutes for 2–3 doses.

Dyspepsia in a bleak, ill-looking, chilly and fussy person. Very poor appetite. May have diarrhoea.

Arsenicum Alb. 6c. One dose at intervals of fifteen to thirty minutes for 2–3 doses.

INFLAMMATION, BOILS AND ABSCESSES

Swelling, pain, tenderness and redness, commonly found on the outer parts of the body, is due to inflammation, and is caused by the defensive reactions of the body to infection by germs. These germs may enter through the damaged skin; in a case of inflammation deep inside the body they may have been carried there by the blood stream. If the defensive reaction is successful the inflammation fades away; but if the reaction is weak, or the infection virulent, an abscess may form.

An abscess is a walled-off collection of pus which is a mixture of liquified dead blood cells, dead germs and nearby tissues. On the surface of the skin it forms the familiar rounded tense mass called a boil. Boils are also frequently formed from the infection of the hair roots.

The natural healing process of an abscess is to form a head and then to discharge the pus. It is safe for a boil on the surface to do this, but it may not be safe for a deep abscess to do so, and antibiotics and surgical help will be needed. If your doctor diagnoses a deep abscess he will refer you to a surgeon; follow his advice. You can also use homoeopathic remedies to good effect at the same time.

A carbuncle is a raised inflamed and infected area of the skin which has several heads or openings, each of which may discharge pus separately. This is a serious condition because it can spread and destroy areas of skin, and can cause a severe general illness. It is also serious because there may be an underlying condition needing diagnosis and treatment, such as diabetes mellitus.

It is essential that you consult your doctor to be investigated. It is almost certain that he will need to give you antibiotics. As above, you should take the appropriate homoeopathic remedies at the same time – there is no risk that they will work against each other.

The required homoeopathic remedies are divided into three groups, relating to the stages of: (i) Inflammation; (ii) Early formation; and (iii) Later formation and discharge of pus. There will tend to be some overlapping, but start at the stage which seems most appropriate, and change the remedy if the picture changes.

Use moist **Hypercal** dressings prepared by adding ten drops to a glass of cool previously boiled water.

INFLAMMATION, BOILS AND ABSCESSES

Inflammation

Early, mild symptoms of inflammation. Slight redness and discomfort. No generalised illness.

Ferrum Phos. 6c. One dose three or four times a day until better.

Skin easily infected. Sharp stabbing pain. Very tender and very sore. Prickling.

Early stage to stop development if possible. **Hepar Sulph. 30c.** One dose every four hours until better.

Later stage to encourage boil to burst. **Hepar Sulph. 6c.** One dose three times a day until better.

Early Formation

As above but also:

Shining and swollen. Pains sting and burn, worse with hot applications and better with cold ones.

Apis Mell. 6c. One dose every one to two hours until better.

Bright red swelling. Hot throbbing pain – worse with cold applications and dressings. Feverish.

Belladonna 6c. One dose every two to three hours until better.

Blue or purple skin around area. Very tender. Worse with hot applications.

Lachesis 6c. One dose every three to four hours until better.

Later Formation and Discharge of Pus

Note all previous remedies.

Hot and cold with chills. Restless, anxious, confused. Rapid pulse and low temperature or high temperature and slow pulse. **Consult your doctor.**

Pyrogen 6c. One dose every two to four hours until better.

Very rapid inflammation. Burning, stinging, throbbing pain. Very tender. Restless and anxious. **Consult your doctor.**

Tarentula Cubensis 30c. One dose every two to four hours until better.

149

INFLUENZA

Influenza is the name given to a very large number of virus infections which usually occur as epidemics, particularly in the cold winter months. It is often found that one or two specific homoeopathic remedies are useful for most of the victims of any particular outbreak.

Prevention is difficult, since the viruses are usually spread by coughs and sneezes in crowded places. However, the use of 'Cold and Flu' tablets (taken one in the morning and evening on the first and perhaps also on the fifteenth of each month) will act like an immunisation and build up the resistance of the patient.

The symptoms vary with each type of virus infection. Usually they divide into those that affect the nose, throat and chest and those that affect the stomach and the bowels. Both groups have general complaints of headaches, muscular aches and pains and fevers. Some viruses can cause bleeding, such as nose bleeds, altered periods, or bruising of the skin (purpura).

The homoeopathic remedies on the page opposite are a few of the main remedies which will help with influenza. Choose the most similar symptom picture. If you cannot decide between two remedies you may give both of them alternately about one hour apart. Watch for changes in the symptoms of the patient and be prepared to change the remedy.

General Measures for Treatment

- For general measures to help the patient see also the Children's Problems section for: 'Colds and Influenza', pages 82–7; 'Fevers', page 98; and in the General Problems section, 'Nausea and Vomiting', page 154; and 'Diarrhoea', page 134.
- Rest the patient, preferably in bed. The room should be warm and ventilated.
- Encourage the patient to drink as much fluid as possible. A light diet is usually preferred by patients – a little and often of what the patient fancies is usually best.

INFLUENZA

First Signs and Early Stages

Fever from cold, dry, frosty weather; cold, dry winds. Red, dry skin. Very thirsty for lots of cold drinks. Anxious, agitated.

Aconite 30c. One dose at intervals of one to two hours for 3–4 doses.

Sudden very high fever. Very red face. Throbbing headache, may be delirious; Hates noise and bright light. May sweat, but usually has hot, *dry* skin.

Belladonna 6c. One dose at intervals of one to two hours and reduce with improvement.

Gradual onset of mild fever. Sweaty skin, pallor and flushing face. May have nosebleeds, earache, and painful tracheitis and cough (i.e. going down into chest).

Ferrum Phos. 6c. One dose two to three times a day.

Later Stages

Red face and throbbing headache. Tired and drowsy; shivering. Aches in back, joint and limbs. Not thirsty.

Gelsemium 6c. One dose every two to three hours until improvement.

Aches and pains and stiffness, helped by restless movements. Sweating in bed – shivering if uncovered. Cold areas of body in spite of fever. Very thirsty for cold drinks. Cold sores in and around mouth (herpes).

Rhus Tox. 6c. One dose every two to three hours until improvement.

Back is sore, stiff and aching. Pain in the eyeballs; muscles and bones ache. Thirsty for cold drinks.

Eupatorium Perfoliatum 6c. One dose at intervals of one to two hours and reduce with improvement.

Sweating. Lies very still because any movement intensifies headache and aches and pains. Very dry mouth and throat. Very great thirst for large drinks of cold water.

Bryonia 6c. One dose at intervals of one to two hours and reduce with improvement.

151

MOUTH ULCERS (APHTHOUS ULCERS)

Most people suffer an occasional ulcer in the mouth, perhaps due to some minor injury from food or a toothbrush bristle. Some people have them in 'crops'. Occasionally, mouth ulcers may persist as a continuous problem for years, one or more developing as the previous one heals. They are very painful and can develop secondary infection. The cause is unknown – orthodox treatments tend to be many and varied, and generally unhelpful to most sufferers.

The homoeopathic remedies on the page opposite should help in the acute stages, and may reduce the severity and frequency of the ulcers. If you only have a few remedies available, Rhus Tox. is likely to be one of them. If the condition is of long standing, or if the remedies do not help, consult a doctor for investigation and assessment. If there is no underlying medical problem, and your attempts at first aid have not been helpful, consult an experienced homoeopath.

MOUTH ULCERS (APHTHOUS ULCERS)

Small red vesicles becoming ulcers. Painful to touch; worse with acid or salty foods.

Borax 6c. One dose three times a day reducing with improvement.

Salivation increased, with metallic taste – but thirsty. Tongue soft and swollen. Bad breath. Shallow ulcers – burning pain. Neck glands may be tender and swollen.

Mercurius Sol. 6c. One dose three times a day, reducing with improvment.

If Merc. Sol. is not effective. Ulcers with irregular edges tending to bleed easily. Stinging, pricking pain.

Nitric Acid 6c. One dose three times a day, reducing with improvement.

Thick, sticky saliva. Tongue swollen. Ulcers especially on inside of lower lip. Cold sores on lower lip.

Hydrastis 6c. One dose three times a day, reducing with improvement.

Tongue red and cracked, or white with a red tip. Gums sore, blisters turning to ulcers. Ulcerated corners of mouth, cold sores on lips.

Rhus Tox. 6c. One dose three times a day, reducing with improvement.

Oral Treatment

Tincture of **Hydrastis** – 20 drops in half a glass of cooled previously boiled water can be used as a mouth wash, as can **Hypercal** or **Calendula** tinctures. Sucking the remedy will also act as local treatment.

NAUSEA AND VOMITING

Everyone is familiar with these symptoms. Nausea may be caused by irritation of the stomach, by infection or overeating and drinking. It may be part of the picture of a particular disease like influenza (page 150) or a condition like pregnancy (page 55). It may be caused by a disturbance of the organ of balance in the ear, as in travel sickness (page 110), or in a specific condition like Menière's disease.

Vomiting occurs when the stomach contents are more or less violently forced up and out of the mouth. Occasionally vomiting occurs suddenly and for no obvious reason, and must then be investigated.

The homoeopathic remedies opposite are a few of a very long list, and should help in most cases.

Care must be taken to prevent dehydration due to vomiting in children, and especially in babies. This is particularly important in very hot weather. Feeding small quantities of water (a little and often), or getting the baby to sip from a teaspoon, should prevent this.

If there is any doubt your doctor should be consulted urgently, or the infant taken to the local hospital.

NAUSEA AND VOMITING

Intense nausea and sweating. No relief from vomiting. Tongue remains clean, profuse saliva. May have diarrhoea also.

Ipecacuanha 6c. One dose at intervals of one to two hours and reduce with improvement.

Burning pain and acid vomiting. Coldness, chills and weakness. Great anxiety. Frequently diarrhoea also.

Arsenicum Alb. 6c. One dose at intervals of one to two hours and reduce with improvement.

No appetite, belching. Tongue coated thick and white. 'Dietary indiscretion' and over-eating. Irritable and complaining.

Antimonium Crud. 6c. One dose at intervals of one to two hours and reduce with improvement.

Bloated, heavy feeling in stomach. Belching, heartburn. 'Dietary indiscretion' and over-eating. Worse in morning and after food. Hypersensitive, irritable, fastidious. 'Morning after the night before'. Hangover.

Nux Vomica 6c. One dose at intervals of one to two hours and reduce with improvement.

OPERATIONS

The effects of surgical operations on most patients are similar, and fairly standard treatments can be offered.

Care Before Operation

Anxiety before admission to hospital, and before operation, can be eased by several remedies. (See also 'Anxiety', page 116.) The three most likely to be helpful are indicated on the opposite page. The remedy chosen can be taken before going to bed for the few nights before going to hospital.

Prevention of Bleeding. Some people bleed readily. Dental and nose and throat operations tend to cause quick bleeding.

Arnica taken before and after the operation tends to reduce bleeding and bruising. For people with a bleeding tendency, or for operations in a region known to bleed freely, Phosphorus is the remedy of choice.

Pain, Bruising and Swelling. These are usual after operations. If Arnica and Hypericum are taken together, before and after the operation, all the unpleasant side effects will be greatly reduced, and far fewer pain-relieving drugs will be required.

Shock. The shock that surgery may produce will be greatly reduced by having taken Arnica beforehand.

There will be no reaction between homoeopathic remedies and the drugs which the hospital medical staff may have to prescribe. When in hospital it is quite possible that the staff will insist that you should not take any other medicines than the ones you are given. This will include homoeopathic remedies. If this is so, there is very little you can do. Please remember that the staff have a legal responsibility for patients in their care, and they must be allowed to conduct treatment as they judge best.

Allergies. Remember to tell the doctors and nurses about known allergies and any adverse reactions you may have had to previous anaesthetics and pain-relieving drugs.

OPERATIONS

Care Before Operation

Anxiety

Anxious. Poor memory. Confused. Weak and trembling. Tendency to diarrhoea.

Gelsemium 30c. One dose for insomnia, and before admission and operation.

Anxiety, excited, agitated. Hurried speech and behaviour. Restless – one unfinished activity after another.

Argentum Nit. 30c. One dose for insomnia, and before admission and operation.

Emotional; oversensitive. Self-centred; changeable moods. Easily distracted from problems. Hysterical behaviour and gestures. Sighing.

Ignatia 30c. One dose a day for a few days before admission.

Prevention of Bleeding

Phosphorus 6c. One dose morning and evening the day before; and one dose the morning of the operation.

Pain, Bruising and Swelling. Shock

Arnica 6c or **30c** and **Hypericum 6c.** One dose of each taken together three times a day the day before operation and continued through the recovery period.

OPERATIONS

Care After Operation

Drowsiness and confusion after the operation are usual in most people for a day or so, but they are more pronounced in some cases. Occasionally this state can last for several days. If this happens (or happened after a previous operation) Opium 30c may be of help, taken on the first day after the operation.

Nausea and vomiting (see page 154).

Bleeding which arises after the operation must obviously be attended to by the surgical and nursing staff, but also take Phosphorus 6c as indicated.

Pain, bruising and swelling will continue to be controlled by taking Arnica 6c and Hypericum 6c.

Flatulence and wind which will not pass either up or down causes painful swelling of the stomach and bowels. If this develops, use Raphanus Niger 6c.

Physical weakness, faintness and general lack of 'get up and go' will be helped by China 6c, three or four times a day, for the first few days after the operation.

'Nervous exhaustion' which develops after operation with some people can be helped by Kali Phos. 30c, three or four times a day for a few days, and then twice a day for about a week as recovery occurs.

OPERATIONS

Care After Operation

Drowsiness, confusion. Especially after a long anaesthetic. Difficulty in waking up.	**Opium 30c.** One dose two or three times on the first day after operation.
Bleeding and oozing of blood.	**Phosphorus 6c.** One dose two or three times on the first day after operation.
Pain, bruising and swelling.	**Arnica 6c** and **Hypericum 6c.** One dose of each together three to four times a day for 3–4 days.
Flatulence, wind. Swelling painful abdomen. Unable to pass wind.	**Raphanus Niger 6c.** One dose at intervals of one to two hours until relief.
Physical weakness. Faintness. Lack of 'get up and go'. Loss of fluids (sweating, bleeding, vomiting).	**China 6c.** One dose four times a day for about one week.
Hypersensitive, irritable, moody. Insomnia. Nervous exhaustion. Weakness. Easily tired. Poor concentration. Unable to get back to work.	**Kali Phos. 30c.** One dose morning and evening for 7–10 days.

PILES (HAEMORRHOIDS)

Piles are veins just inside the anus which begin to bulge and enlarge, and eventually to extrude or 'prolapse'. Initially the extruded or prolapsed piles return on their own, but they may eventually need to be pushed back after each motion has passed.

In Western countries the main cause of piles in both men and women is likely to be the low fibre content of the diet, causing some degree of constipation, although a bout of severe diarrhoea may also produce piles. A particular cause in women is the pressure of a baby during pregnancy and the force of straining in confinement. There can also be a family tendency to have piles.

The treatment of piles must be based on a diet containing adequate roughage, and this is best obtained from natural and unrefined foods. Sometimes an increase in liquids is needed as well.

Use the appropriate homoeopathic remedy. If the piles are prolapsed and painful the use of liquid paraffin (medicinal paraffin) for a few days can be helpful in softening the individual motions. The dose varies with the patient, but it is useful to start with one teaspoonful with the main meals and vary according to the results. *Do not continue the use of medicinal paraffin for more than one or two weeks.*

Caution

If you have used suitably chosen remedies and improved your diet and bowel habit over a month or two, and there has still been no improvement with the piles, or if they seem to be worse, consult a doctor.

But if the piles suddenly appear for no very obvious reason, or if they gradually enlarge, protrude and bleed, or if you develop a change of bowel habit, or at any time pass blood or mucus with the motions, **then you must consult your doctor immediately**. He will assess the situation, and decide if investigations are needed to exclude any serious disease, and what other methods of treatment ought to be considered.

PILES (HAEMORRHOIDS)

Constipation, or a loose early morning motion. Anal itching. Fullness, little bleeding. Headache and constipation.

Sulphur 6c. One dose morning and evening and reduce with improvement.

Piles: large, burning and stinging. Worse at night. Irritability. Constipated, small stools and a 'never finished' feeling.

Nux Vomica 6c. One dose each night and reduce with improvement.

Piles: protruding like grapes. Bleeding. Scraped, burning sensation. Better for bathing with cold water.

Aloes 6c. One dose three times a day and reduce with improvement.

Piles: purple and bruised-looking. Splinter-like feeling in rectum. Anus dry, itching and burning. Low back pain.

Aesculus 6c. One dose three times a day and reduce with improvement.

It can be very difficult to decide which remedy is most likely to be effective, and indeed there are several others possible. In this case take Nux Vomica 6c at night on retiring and Sulphur 6c first thing in the morning for one or two weeks.

External Treatment

Apply one or other of the following ointments night and morning, or after each motion: **Hamamelis**, **Aesculus** or **Paeonia** (see page 176 under 'Ointments and Creams'). Although it is sometimes very difficult to do, washing after each bowel action helps to control itching and soreness. A spray bidet can be especially helpful.

PSORIASIS

This is the name given to a long-term skin condition which may arise in childhood, although usually later, with patches of thickening skin, crusting and scaling, and sometimes cracking and bleeding fissures.

It can occur on any area of the skin, but is typically found on the knees, elbows and in the scalp. Great thickness of the skin is typical of the elbows and knees, sometimes with cracking and bleeding. The scalp is more usually the site of great scaling, like severe 'dandruff'.

Psoriasis tends to run in families, and sometimes seems to be brought about by excessive anxiety and stress. If this is thought to play a part, it is important to consult a homoeopath, because a thorough assessment of the family background and the psychological and physical make-up of the patient will be essential. Even so, treatment is likely to take several months.

ROSACEA (ACNE ROSACEA)

This is an abnormal reaction of the skin of the face, which eventually gives rise to a reddening and thickening of the skin. It covers the cheeks and sometimes the forehead. There is initially a variable flushing which gradually becomes more constant, with later prominent blood vessels, and later still, red, thickened skin and small spots.

There is frequently a sensation of burning and stinging, which is intensified by hot drinks and alcohol. It is most frequent in women at the menopause, but can occur in alcoholics of either sex. Rosacea is particularly disturbing since it so often comes with all the other problems of the menopausal age.

If the patient is very disturbed psychologically, if the suggested remedies provide insufficient relief, consult an experienced homoeopath, who will ensure that the constitutional homoeopathic treatment is given.

PSORIASIS

Fine, dry, scaling patches of skin. Burning, itching improved by local warmth.

Arsenicum Alb. 6c. One dose morning and evening.

Blood-stained fissures and cracks in very thickened skin patches. Itching not relieved by scratching.

Sepia 6c. One dose morning and evening.

Leathery skin with rough, thickened and cracking patches. Nails thickened, splitting and pitted. Worse in winter.

Petroleum 6c. One dose morning and evening.

ROSACEA (ACNE ROSACEA)

Red, flushed skin. Granular appearance. Enlarged veins. Very symmetrical areas on cheeks and central forehead.

Arnica 6c. One dose a day.

Red, burning, stinging areas on the cheeks made worse by local heat. Hot flushes with red cheeks.

Sanguinaria Canadensis 6c. One dose morning and evening.

The treatment may have to be continued for several weeks.

External Treatment

This should be gentle. On no account should ointments or creams containing cortisone-type drugs be used. Applications of **Hamamelis** cream may be used, depending upon the individual response.

SHINGLES (HERPES ZOSTER)

This is a very painful skin rash which follows the route of a nerve in the skin, and is caused by the chickenpox virus. The skin becomes inflamed, painful and tender so that movement, and even the touch of clothes, is intolerable. The variably-sized areas of inflammation develop several types of blisters which then burst and form dry scabs. Any area of the body surface can be affected. The head and face can be particularly troublesome.

If the eye is affected you must consult your own doctor. He will probably refer you to an eye specialist.

The aching or neuralgic shooting pains usually start before the skin rash appears, which can give rise to difficulties in diagnosis. If there is any doubt your family doctor should be consulted.

During all this time the patient is usually very unwell, with general aches, pains, malaise and some fever, and may have to go to bed.

General Treatment

- Stay off work.
- Bed rest is usually needed in the early stages, although some people may feel better for being up and about.
- The skin may have to be protected from contact with clothes. This can best be done by covering it with cottonwool pads held in position by either sticking plaster or crepe bandages, but movement makes it difficult to keep these in place for long. Some patients find Calendula ointment spread on sterile dressings very soothing, although if this is kept in position too long the skin may become soggy.
- The oozing from the blisters can be dressed by placing Melolin dressings over each area. Melolin is less likely to stick to the skin and absorbs the discharge.
- Oozing in the beard, scalp and hairy skin is best not dressed, but left alone for as long as possible. Sponging with a solution of Calendula or Hypercal tincture may help, twenty drops to half a pint of cool, previously boiled water.
- Try to reduce the pain by covering or applying hot or cold compresses to the shingles. Sometimes keeping very still (or moving about) will help the pain. If you find out what can improve (or worsen) the pain, this will help you to choose a remedy.

SHINGLES (HERPES ZOSTER)

Early treatment is important if severe neuralgic pains are to be prevented or reduced. The appearance of the rash and the things which aggravate or relieve the pain are of importance in choosing the remedy. If you find that your pain is not helped by your choice of remedy, alternate the two most likely remedies.

Very small blisters with clear fluid. Pain and itching helped by restless movement. Hot compresses may relieve the pain.

Rhus Tox. 6c. One dose four times a day while the blisters last.

Severe itching, burning pain, may be worse after midnight. Pain relieved by hot compresses. Restless, anxious, sleepless.

Arsenicum Alb. 6c. One dose four times a day while the blisters last.

Large blisters with surrounding swelling. Burns, stings, prickles. Relieved by cool compresses.

Apis 6c. One dose four times a day while the blisters last.

Bluish blisters with bloodstained fluid. Itching. Touch and movement causes shocks and stabs of pain. Pain reduced by stillness and rest.

Ranunculus Bulbosus 6c. One dose four times a day while the blisters last.

If your first-aid treatment has not proved effective within a week, consult an experienced homoeopath without further delay.

TOOTHACHE

What we usually call toothache may have many causes, but it is usually due to 'bad teeth', and for that the cure is to visit the dentist.

There are many types of pain and many factors, such as the position of the pain, the alteration of the severity by hot or cold drinks or foods, and the effect of eating, pressure or touch.

If there is throbbing, swelling of the gum or face, a rise in temperature and a general feeling of being unwell, there is likely to be an infection. There may also be an abscess forming, described variously as a dental abscess, a root abscess or a gum boil. (See also 'Dental Abscess', page 132.)

The list of possible remedies is much larger than shown here, but one among the selection on the page opposite may help you until the dentist can deal with the problem.

N.B. Remember to use **Arnica 6c** with or without **Hypericum 6c** before and after dental treatment.

TOOTHACHE

Stabbing, shooting pain. 'Neuralgia'. Brought on by ice cream or very cold winds, or iced drinks.

Aconite 6c. One dose every fifteen minutes for 6–8 doses.

Teeth extremely sensitive to touch and feel long. Profuse salivation.

Plantago 6c. One dose every fifteen minutes for 6–8 doses.

Painful local swelling near tooth. Stabbing pain to the ear. Teeth feel loose and tender. Thirst with increased salivation.

Mercurius Sol. 6c. One dose every hour for 6–8 hours.

Local throbbing pain of a gum boil, with much swelling of the face and mouth.

Apis 6c. One dose every hour.

Apis and Mercurius Sol. 6c can be taken alternately every hour for several doses.

Obvious bad teeth but no gum boil. Bad breath and bitter taste.

Kreosote 6c. One dose every hour.

Pain – drawing and tearing. Teeth very sensitive to touch or cold air. Worse at night and after food. Cheek may be swollen and red. Patient irritable and resentful.

Staphysagria 6c. One dose every fifteen minutes for 6–8 doses.

Patient is intolerant, restless and peevish with the severe pain. Worse at night. Worse with warm food or drinks.

Chamomilla 6c. One dose every fifteen minutes for 6–8 doses.

A Basic Materia Medica

In the first part of this book, the illness or injury itself is discussed, together with the different groups of symptoms that indicate which particular homoeopathic remedies are likely to be needed to treat the individual patients.

What follows in the next few pages is a list of homoeopathic remedies, together with a brief description of the diseases and conditions which might be helped by each one. Each description of a remedy involves the sorts of minor ailments that can reasonably be treated at home, and at the same time begins to build up a description of the 'properties' of the remedy.

The 'properties' or 'characteristics' of a remedy relate to the kind of physical and emotional symptoms that recur in any individual's life, and to the particular external and emotional circumstances that affect their well-being, either positively or adversely. It is found that amongst the major homoeopathic remedies there will be one which is of special value to the person who corresponds more or less to such a 'symptom picture'. The remedy is thus directly relevant to that individual's constitution, and such remedies are known as 'constitutional remedies'.

The short remedy-pictures that follow are only outline descriptions of some of the important constitutional remedies in homoeopathy. If you wish to extend your knowledge of the remedies, especially the emotional and more general characteristics, there are several books which you might find helpful. There is a book list on page 180. I have deliberately not gone into these aspects of the remedies in the brief sketches below, because I do not think it helps the particular purpose of this book, which is First-Aid.

Aconite

SHOCK—CROUP—FRIGHT—FEVER—ACCIDENTS—CHILLS

The beginning of colds, 'flu', fevers – especially if restless, anxious, thirsty or severely chilled.

In emergencies like accidents, bereavements, animal or insect bites, asthma or bleeding, especially if distressed with fear, palpitations of the heart, breathlessness, trembling and numbness and tingling of the face and fingers.

Antimonium Crudum

UPSET STOMACH

No appetite with belching, bloated stomach, thick white coated tongue, cracked corners of the mouth.

Depressed and irritable. Baby vomits feeds.

Sick headaches from thick catarrh, too much alcohol, bathing.

Feels better with acid drinks or pickles.

Antimonium Tartaricum

COUGH

Wheezing bronchitis, rattling cough, difficult to get the phlegm up.

Breathless, suffocating, gasping, must sit up to get ease.

Pale faced, weak, clammy cold skin.

Arnica

INJURY

If shocked, give Aconite first.

Bruising, sprains, concussion, accidents, operations.

Aching muscles from overuse in work or sports.

Before and after dental surgery (with Hypericum).

Overtiredness.

Arsenicum Album

VOMITING AND DIARRHOEA—FOOD POISONING—'GASTRIC FLU'

Especially when vomiting and diarrhoea occur together.

Very chilly, anxious, restless, weak.

Burning pains in the stomach. Thirst – likes warm drinks.

Nauseated by sight and smell of food.

Belladonna

HIGH FEVER—THROBBING—SORE THROAT—SUNSTROKE—HEADACHE—EARACHE—BOILS

Very red cheeks, pale around the lips.

Wide open eyes, wide open pupils.

Excited, perhaps delirious. Thirsty but won't drink during a fever.

Very hot, dry skin, perhaps a scarlet rash.

Bryonia

PAINS—BURSTING HEADACHE

Arthritis, Pleurisy, Migraine.

Pains worse from movement, breathing, warmth.

Pains better for lying still, pressure, cool.

The patient is *very* thirsty for cold drinks.

Camphor

Note: Camphor should always be kept separate from other homoeopathic remedies as it may inactivate them.

CHILLS

Feels better for warmth.

First signs of a cold when chilled and sneezing.

Diarrhoea from a chill – 'feels frozen'.

Cantharis

CYSTITIS—BURNS AND SCALDS—BLISTERS—GNAT BITES

Cystitis – scalding, burning urine which may be blood-stained, passed in drops. Pain before, during and after urination. Painful urging. Frequency.

Burns and scalds – pain eased with cold applications.

Carbo Vegetabilis

WIND—FLATULENCE—COLLAPSE

Stomach distended and belching wind. Relieved by sitting up and loosening clothes. General physical collapse with skin pale or bluish. Pulseless. Cold, cold sweat. Gasping for fresh air and feels better if the face is fanned and propped up.

Chamomilla

UNBEARABLE PAIN. Frantic child with EARACHE, TOOTHACHE, TEETHING, COLIC

A child may be pacified by being picked up but may remain very difficult, irritable and angry. One cheek may be red and hot.

Generally may be made worse by bouts of anger.

Green diarrhoea may accompany the colic.

Colocynthis

COLIC—NEURALGIC PAIN—GRIPING PAIN

Three-month colic in babies.

Abdominal colic eased by bending over, firm pressure or a hot water bottle.

Griping pains distended with wind, belching, vomiting.

Colic or neuralgia from anger, resentment or becoming worked up.

Euphrasia

HAY FEVER—MEASLES

Measles, early stage with streaming tears that burn, light that hurts, head throbs.

Sneezing, running nose, cough.

Hay fever with similar symptoms, made worse indoors, in the evenings or in warm weather.

Gelsemium

INFLUENZA—HEADACHE—ANXIETY—SORE THROAT

Influenza – drowsy, 'drugged' feeling. Weakness.

Aching, shivery back.

Aching, trembling limbs.

'Thick head' – aching back of head, neck, heavy-eyed.

Sneezing, running nose, sore throat and painful swallowing. Not thirsty.

Anxiety – Especially *before* an event or difficult situation.

Hepar Sulphuris

BOILS—ABSCESSES—INFECTED SPOTS—TONSILLITIS—COUGH

Tonsillitis with splinter-like pains (sometimes into the ear).

Cough dry and deep with tightness of the chest or cough with wheezing and rattling chest.

Patients can be irritable, oversensitive, discontented, grumbling and impetuous. They usually feel better in warm, wet weather, but their problems can be made worse by touch or cold draught.

Hypericum

WOUNDS OR OPERATIONS—PAINFUL INJURIES TO NERVES OF FINGERS, TOES, NAILS, LIPS, GUMS AND TEETH

Any sort of injury where the nerve endings have been damaged, causing severe pain and sensitivity.

Before and after dental treatment or operations.

Ipecacuanha

NAUSEA—COUGH

Continuous nausea with no relief from vomiting. Clean tongue and too much saliva.

Cough with congested wheezing chest. Nosebleeds and other haemorrhages with nausea.

Mercurius Solubilis

FEVERISH COLDS—ULCERATED MOUTH AND THROAT

Offensive-smelling sweat, breath or mucus.

Generally weak and trembling.

Feels chilly in the cold, too hot in the warmth.

Greatly increased saliva but very thirsty.

Profuse yellow, green catarrh.

Diarrhoea persisting with painful straining, slime and perhaps blood.

Worse at night and in the warmth.

Natrum Muriaticum

SNEEZING—COLDS—COLD SORES

Profuse watery nasal catarrh with sneezing.

Generally chilly but worse in a warm room.

Greasy skin, likes salt, thirsty.

Weary, weepy and irritable. Effects of grief.

Nux Vomica

UPSET STOMACH—INDIGESTION—INFLUENZA—HEADACHE

Indigestion from too much food or alcohol. Belching bitter fluid. Bloated 'heavy weight' feeling hours after eating. Hangover.

Nausea, constipation or frequent unsatisfactory bowel movements. Itching piles.

'Stuffy' cold with dry blocked nose, worse in the open air, improving in a warm room. Very irritable. Sensitive. Reproachful.

Influenza, with a very chilled feeling.

Phosphorus

LARYNGITIS—REPEATED VOMITING—BLEEDING

Nosebleeds. Bleeding after dental extractions.

Hoarse voice, painful talking, chest tight.

Loss of voice.

Cough – dry, tickling, racking made worse by moving out into cold air. Made worse by talking.

Gastritis – wants cold drinks but soon vomits them back.

Pulsatilla

CATARRH—MEASLES—INDIGESTION

Catarrh – yellow-green of eye, nose.

Loss of sense of smell.

Dry mouth but *not* thirsty.

Loose cough worse in a warm room.

Measles – catarrhal stage with a greeny-yellow nasal catarrh.

Indigestion from fatty, oily or rich foods.

Generally feels much better in fresh air.

Rhus Toxicodendron

ARTHRITIS—FIBROSITIS—RHEUMATISM—SHINGLES—SPRAINS

Pains and stiffness – worse in cold, wet weather, cold air, after rest, on getting up from a chair or out of bed.

First movements painful and stiff – keeping moving eases the pain and stiffness.

Influenza with rheumaticky pains and stiffness and a dry cough.

Itching, tender blisters and rash. Mouth ulcers and cold sores.

Sulphur

SKIN RASHES

Burning, itching skin rashes. Eczema.

Worse for heat of bed, scratching, bathing and clothes.

Boils, styes, piles – burning pain.

Morning diarrhoea.

To conclude treatment for infections and inflammations.

The 'Medicine Chest'

The domestic 'medicine chest' for homoeopathic medicines is really a container for all the remedies which have accumulated over a period of time. It can be any convenient box or tin. In contrast to ordinary medicines, it is quite safe to keep homoeopathic remedies for future use.

Some homoeopathic pharmacists still dispense remedies in the traditional 7 gram glass tubes and sell boxes containing compartments for each tube. Others dispense in either glass or plastic containers of differing sizes. It is useful to write the names of the remedy and the potency on a circular label on the plastic screw top. Another useful tip is to print a sheet of card in the top of the box as an alphabetical list of each remedy with the potency.

A basic list of remedies follows, together with an extended list.

As you treat yourself and the family you will use a variety of remedies, and some tablets or pills will be left over. Keep them – do not throw them away, because in this way you will build up your medicine chest. They will reflect the common problems of your family and will be readily to hand if needed.

BASIC LIST OF HOMOEOPATHIC REMEDIES FOR STARTING THE MEDICINE CHEST

Aconite	Belladonna	Natrum Mur.
Antimonium Crud.	Bryonia	Nux Vomica
Antimonium Tart.	Chamomilla	Phosphorus
Arnica	Ipecacuanha	
Arsenicum Alb.	Mercurius Sol.	

EXTENDED LIST OF HOMOEOPATHIC REMEDIES

Allium Cepa	Euphrasia	Lycopodium
Apis Mel.	Ferrum Phos.	Pulsatilla
Argentum Nit.	Gelsemium	Rhus Tox.
Cantharis	Hamamelis	Ruta
Carbo Veg.	Hepar Sulph.	Sepia
Cocculus	Hypericum	Spongia
Colocynthis	Ignatia	Sulphur
Drosera	Ledum	Urtica

SOME HOMOEOPATHIC OINTMENTS AND CREAMS

Aesculus – swollen, prolapsing piles.

Arnica – for bruising (but *not* with broken skin).

Calendula – for cuts and grazes; antiseptic effect; stimulates the healing process

Graphites – skin problems, especially when broken and oozing clear fluid.

Hamamelis – for bruising with broken skin; bleeding piles.

Hypericum – crushed nerve endings; bed sores; can be made up in a bland oil.

Paeonia – unbearable itching: piles and anus, vulvae, skin.

Rhus Tox. – joints which are stiff in cold, damp weather.

Ruta – sprains and strains; internal damage.

Tamus – chilblains.

Urtica Urens – burns and sunburn; stinging eczema; itching vulvae; nettle rash (urticaria).

TINCTURES

Arnica – for bruising.

Calendula – for grazes and wounds.

'Hypercal' – for grazes and wounds. This is a mixture of the tinctures of Hypericum and Calendula.

Urtica Urens – for burns or itching.

The First Aid Box

It is useful and more efficient to have First Aid items together in a suitably marked box which is always kept in the same place.

Personal preference plays a large part in what you have in it, but the following list may be a useful guide to begin with.

1) Adhesive plasters, assorted sizes.
2) Adhesive plaster, one roll. (Remember that some people may be allergic to certain types of plaster.)
3) Cotton wool, one sterilised small pack.
4) Wound dressing, sterilised and *non*-medicated. Small, medium and large, two of each.
5) Gauze squares, sterilised and *non*-medicated, one pack.
6) Gauze bandages, sterilised and *non*-medicated, assorted sizes.
7) Eye pad, sterilised and with tapes.
8) Crepe bandage, 3 inch width.
9) Small round-ended scissors.
10) Tweezers for applying dressings.

Organisations Concerned With Homoeopathy

The following organisations will send books, publications and information on where homoeopathic treatment may be obtained in your area, as well as the addresses of the pharmacists who can supply homoeopathic remedies. It would be appreciated if you wrote to them in the first instance enclosing a stamped, addressed envelope.

The Faculty of Homoeopathy, The Royal London Homoeopathic Hospital, Great Ormond Street, London WC1N 3HR, Tel: 01-837 3091, Ext. 85 or 72

Membership of the Faculty is only open to doctors medically qualified in the United Kingdom, or in countries and medical schools recognised by the General Medical Council. Members and Fellows have all received postgraduate training in homoeopathic medicine and passed the examination of the Faculty. They use the letters MFHom after their other degrees and qualifications.

The British Homoeopathic Association, 27a Devonshire Street, London WC1N 1RJ, Tel: 01-935 2163.

The Hahnemann Society, Humane Education Centre, Avenue Lodge, Bounds Green Road, London N22 4EU, Tel: 01-889 1595.

Homoeopathic Development Foundation, 19a Cavendish Square, London W1M 9AD, Tel: 01-629 3205.

Any general practitioner working as a family doctor in the National Health Service is able to refer his patients to the Outpatients Department of the following NHS homoeopathic hospitals, for consultation with consultant homoeopathic physicians.

The Royal London Homoeopathic Hospital, Great Ormond Street, London WC1N 3HR. Tel: 01-837 8833 (Appointments 01-837 7821).

Glasgow Homoeopathic Hospital, 100 Great Western Road, Glasgow
G12 0RN. Tel: 041-339 0382.

Bristol Homoeopathic Hospital, Cotham Road, Cotham, Bristol BS6 6JU.
Tel: 0272-731231.

Tunbridge Wells Homoeopathic Hospital, Church Road, Tunbridge Wells,
Kent TN1 1JU. Tel: 0892-42977.

Department of Homoeopathic Medicine, Mossley Hill Hospital,
Park Avenue, Liverpool L18 8BU. Tel: 051-724 2335.

In addition to homoeopathic doctors, there are professional homoeopathic
practitioners who are not doctors. These homoeopaths will have studied
the subject in a variety of ways and for variable lengths of time. They are
permitted to advertise, whereas doctors are not.

The Society of Homoeopaths issues a register of those practitioners
whom it recognises as being qualified and competent to practise. For a
copy of this register you may contact: The Secretary, The Society of
Homoeopaths, 47 Canada Grove, Bognor Regis, West Sussex PO21 1DW.
Tel: 0243-860678.

Books Recommended for Further Study

Homoeopathic Prescribing, by Dr Noel Pratt, Beaconsfield Publishers.

This book deals with many more problems than *Everyday Homoeopathy*, but the remedy descriptions are usually brief and this may be difficult for the beginner. The outline descriptions of the more important constitutional remedies introduce the idea of the patient's total constitutional picture in a basic way, and this is helpful. Also helpful is the interleaving of blank pages for note-making and observations.

Decachords, by A. Gladstone Clarke, Missionary School of Medicine, 2 Powis Place, London WC1N 3HT.

Basic constitutional descriptions for a larger number of homoeopathic remedies.

Introduction to Homoeopathic Medicine, by Dr Hamish Boyd, Beaconsfield Publishers.

This book gives systematic instruction in the basics of all aspects of homoeopathic medicine. While not ordinarily needed in the home, it is a very useful book for those wishing to study homoeopathy in more detail.

Important Telephone Numbers

General Practitioner:

Homoeopath:

Dentist:

District Nurse:

Midwife:

Health Visitor:

Ambulance – In Emergency Only – Dial 999

Homoeopathic Pharmacy:

Acupuncturist:

Chiropractor:

Osteopath:

Others:

Index of Problems